I0415384

The Highs & Lows of My Infertility

A Collection of Personal Blog Posts from IVF to Surrogacy

Bianca Smith

DEDICATION

Dedicated to all the LOVE in my life. Especially my incredible sons,
Maximus Vincent & Alexei Felix & their equally amazing dad, Vinny.

Cover design by Jo from https://cosmic-creations.co.za

For more information on the author visit

https://wheresmystork.com

Also by the same author

IVF A Detailed Guide: Everything I wish I Had Known Before Starting My Fertility Treatments

available on Amazon Kindle, Paperback & AUDIO

My Ukrainian Surrogacy Journey

A Personal Account of My Mission to Motherhood in Kiev

Available on Amazon Kindle & Paperback

The Highs & Lows of My Infertility

Hi Friends!

Welcome to snippets of one of the most challenging times of my life –
trying to fulfil my life's destiny of becoming a mom. My story doesn't
start at the beginning – there is no beginning. From the time I was a
little girl playing with all my kids (my dolls) – feeding them, burping
them, changing them, shopping & cooking for them and even home-
schooling them, I looked forward to growing up and having my own
family to love and take care of.

This book doesn't start at the beginning of that, nor does it start at the
point where depression took over my life at the realisation that
procreating naturally was never written for me.

This book starts in the middle of my IVF treatments. *Why?* Because
somewhere in the middle of one of my lowest dips on the fertility
rollercoaster is when I decided that the weight of dealing with fertility
challenges was too much to carry on my own. It was dragging me down
into a dark hole and the only way I was going to stop myself from
getting swallowed whole by this black pit, was going to be by writing
down my feelings and throwing them out into the world as a form of
self-medicating.

My online blog, *Where's My stork?* was born in 2015. My first intentions
with my blog was a place to vent. A place to describe how terrible my

life was for being handed this burden. A place to sob in despair one minute and be angry at the world the next minute, while gathering a tribe by my side who could be just as sad or angry with me – to help me carry the burden.

However, *Where's My Stork?* took on a life form and direction of its own. Before I knew it, my blog morphed into a source of encouragement and inspiration first to myself and then to many others. I received a ton of emails from readers telling me how some days my blog messages were all that got them through that day after yet another negative pregnancy test or experiencing another miscarriage. I also received messages from readers who had no fertility issues but felt encouraged by my words in other areas of their lives. This wasn't something planned – it just happened. While I have always firmly believed that motherhood was my destiny, it seems like all my years and hardships on the fertility rollercoaster has also been part of my destiny so that my story can be shared to give others a feeling of camaraderie, hope, realism and encouragement to keep going despite the setbacks, and to look at life from a new perspective.

This book is a collection of all my personal blog posts – every raw emotion and experience that I documented about my fertility experiences. Each piece is written based on exactly how I felt at those times – my soul laid bare.

My first fertility book, IVF A Detailed Guide, is information regarding procedures, processes, embryos, tests, etc presented in terms that people like me who are not in the medical field can relate to. All the information in the books was verified by fertility experts but it is written for you and me going through IVF and not having a clue what's going on at the start of our journeys. As the subtitle, says, it really is everything I wish I had known before starting my fertility journey. What you won't find in this book is my personal story. It's factual and not emotional.

My second fertility book, My Ukrainian Surrogacy Story, is a guide for those who are interested in pursuing surrogacy. It describes why we chose Ukraine, what we did to prepare for surrogacy, our exact uncensored experiences with the agency/clinic used and all the legal paperwork we as British citizens needed to gather, prepare and submit to governmental authorities. My surrogacy book is written based on personal experiences and expectations, but the focus is on the surrogacy journey.

This book in your hands, the third and last of my fertility books, is literally my raw diary entries from my blog with flaws, vulnerabilities, disappointments, celebrations and everything in between.

My *Where's My Stork?* website is taking on a different direction now. It will embark on a process of changing from a personal story to an informational hub. One of the reasons I wanted to put this book together, is for my journey to be remembered by the people that matter most to me in a keepsake instead of it just disappearing off my website – a personal keepsake for me and mine and also, I hope for it to be a book of encouragement for those going through not only fertility but any other challenges in life.

Thank you always to my tribe, supporters and readers for keeping my strength and spirits up over the years.

With love,
Bianca

My First Blog Entry of My First Online Diary
Hello & Welcome to Where's My Stork?
Published by Bianca on 30 March 2015

First a look at the very beginning of my Fertility Story

In 2005 I got married at 29 years old full of hopes and dreams to start a big family. One year on, me and my *then* husband still struggled to conceive. Professionals advised me that I had a condition called Grave's Disease, which is an extremely overactive thyroid. Plus, I was told that I had PCOS (Polycystic Ovarian Syndrome), where one doesn't actually release the egg down the fallopian tube but the egg turns into a cyst, preventing normal ovulation and thus fertilisation and conception – a condition suffered by more than 10,000,000 women worldwide.

For treatment, I was given Clomid (Fertomid in South Africa) to stimulate ovulation) Metformin (Glucophage in South Africa) to counteract the weight gain from the Clomid, and Carbimazole (to reduce the production of the thyroid hormones, thyroxine). Over the next 6 months, this combination of meds made me extremely ill – my weight rapidly decreased from a UK size 10 to child size (smaller than a UK size 6), I suffered from leg cramps on a daily basis, so bad that I couldn't function day or night. I would wake up in the middle of the night screaming in pain and my (now ex) husband would have to spend a few hours trying to massage the cramps. I would get sudden cramping attacks at work and would need to either lie down on the back-office floor while a colleague would have to try and massage the cramps or I would need to pace up and down, moving my legs in different directions. I couldn't travel far at any time as being in one position for too long would make things worse. I was on all sorts of prescribed cramp blockers and was the subject of many medical discussions. No one could quite work out where these attacks had suddenly come from and why nothing would take them away.

Everyone was baffled. To me, it seemed obvious that it must have something to do with the medication I was on. The doctors did not want to take me off the medication and threatened that it could be detrimental to my health to stop them. Really??? I never went back to the doctors. I took myself off the destructive medicinal cocktail. The cramps stopped a few months after that.

My then husband and I decided to pursue IVF – in a nutshell......he was a workaholic, hardly ever at home, could never make doctor's appointments and so the IVF never seemed to get started. After about 9 months of depression and frustration on my side (over not conceiving as well as several other marital issues) I ended the marriage.

What followed was a long period of self-loathing coupled with self-destructive habits that I won't discuss here but you're welcome to take your imagination to a dark place.

Then, I moved from South Africa to the UK, met my soul mate a year later and warned him from the get-go that I was probably not capable of having kids, so he needed to think long and hard whether he wanted to continue in a relationship with me or not. Lucky for me, he wasn't going to let that stop him.

Between then and writing this entry, it has been a hell of a journey already!! Very few couples have been through the amount of trials and heartache that we have been through from almost the start of being together.

At the end of 2010, we found out by accident that we had a chemical pregnancy. This is when an egg and sperm fertilise and the embryo tries to burrow in and attach but doesn't quite get a grip. The egg falls and is expelled from the body early on, long before any heartbeat can be seen on a scan. In fact, doctors say that a large percentage of women have repeated chemical pregnancies and never realise it, thinking they are just having heavy periods.

After discovering that we were so close to having a family, we cried and tended to broken hearts and then something awakened in us. An ever-increasing yearning for a family of our own. We went to the GP to start the fertility treatment process.

Things happen very slowly in the world of the NHS (National Health Service) in the UK and it took another 2.5 years before the treatments started. First it was my thyroid again. I couldn't escape taking meds for my thyroid any longer, especially as the doctors led me to believe that my fertility struggles were probably from my over active thyroid. After some tweaking, we found a treatment that didn't make me sick (Propylthiouracil –

PTU). My endocrinologist was convinced that I would be pregnant within 6 months of this thyroid treatment, as most of her patients had been. She's still currently baffled, wondering why I'm not pregnant.

And my PCOS? A series of scans and second and third and fourth opinions revealed that I had no PCOS (I subsequently have learnt that PCOS can come and go sporadically throughout a woman's 'fertile' years. Ok great, so once my thyroid was balanced, I would conceive, I thought. Wrong - 6 months came and went, another 3 months came and went. Still no pregnancy. The wolves of depression snarled at my door and it took everything my hubby and I had not to lose each other in a black hole of misery. Living through this was tough. Next began a series of blood tests, which, in typical NHS (non)competence, were repeated several times. Everything appeared to be normal. No problem could be found with my womb. No problem with my ovaries. No problem with ovulating. I did a hysterosalpingogram (HSG), which is where they shoot dye through the tubes to check for blockages – and, well, you guessed it…everything normal.

Finally, we were sent to an IVF coordinator who sat in a chair opposite me and told me that I had something called unexplained infertility (stinging words for anyone with fertility problems – ***unexplained***!! Most people with this non-condition (for lack of a better way to describe it) would give a lot to rather have an explained condition. When you have a problem and someone has identified it, you are already halfway to fixing the problem. And if it can't be fixed, it's easier (I can only imagine – I could be wrong) to accept, than having no explanation! How do you fix an unexplained problem?!?

So, there I sat feeling like me and my unexplained problem would at least finally be getting somewhere because in front of me was an IVF coordinator who confirmed that she was referring us to do IVF (over a year since making enquiries). Also, due to my age (wrong side of my 30's) and the fact that we both didn't have any children, and that we had been trying for so long with no success, and that we lived in the 'right area' (the UK has this postcode lottery when it comes to government subsidised rounds of IVF), we would be eligible for 3 free IVF cycles and would be moved up to the top of the waiting list. Whoop! Whoop! Hooray! I wanted to dance with happiness right there in her office. That was until she told me the catch – we would be contacted by the IVF nurses in 6 months' time and be given our referral to the fertility clinic. What?! So, all the tests had been done (several times) and all the powers that be had confirmed that we were eligible to be referred for IVF, but we had to wait another 6 months to even meet with the clinic!! Heart wrenching!

6 Intense, frustrating, teary, depressing months later – to the day – I called the IVF coordinator to demand my referral. Guess what? The test results (the same tests that I had done several times already) had now expired and I had to re-do them! Did someone say Groundhog Day?!

At last, in June 2013, we met with the IVF nurses at our referred fertility clinic and planned our first IVF cycle. I started the meds on 11 July 2013 and was absolutely amazed to discover that our IVF had worked!!! And first time too!!! On Saturday 5 October at 4am, I saw those two heavenly lines on the pee stick given to me 12 days before by the clinic. This was one of the happiest days of my life, ever! Ever! I will never forget any moment – how I sat, how I felt, how I jumped on the bed to give Vinny the news, what we did afterwards, how we celebrated and how complete I felt. Two weeks later my scan showed one little baby with a healthy flickering heartbeat.

On 25 November 2013 at my 12-week scan, filled with so much excitement, we were stunned to discover that our baby's heartbeat had in fact stopped somewhere between 7 and 8 weeks. It was a missed-miscarriage or alternatively called a silent miscarriage due to no blood loss to tell me that the baby was gone. He or she was still there, only not alive. I will never be able to describe that feeling of utter despair and disbelief. We were broken.

There was a glimmer of hope, a silver lining in that stormy darkness – the fact that IVF had worked for me. This meant that there was absolutely no doubt that cycle number 2 was going to give us our take home baby.

But it was not to be.

And neither was cycle number 3, 4 or 5.

And here we are now…THE CURRENT STORY

I've just spent a few weeks filled with tears and rage of volcanic proportions, fuelled by heavy doses of oestrogen, progesterone, a 5th failed IVF cycle, stinking cold that won't leave, a bleeding ulcer that just won't subside (I expect from all the medication I'm on) and sexual frustration (sadly, normal sex is banned during most of each IVF cycle).

Don't worry, this week I have made a comeback. The hubby and I had a catch up (*wink* * wink*) – although that's a short-lived one-time only session until after the next cycle (yes, IVF is extremely romantic blah! Right?!). I am focused and excited on IVF nr 6 happening soon. I am off the horrid progesterone for two weeks (although still on the oestrogen – much to my husband's displeasure, as the side effects make things a bit more than a little windy! How attractive! Ha ha! Something like a whirlwind hovering over a sewer – you get the pretty picture I'm sure :-)).

In the depth of the explosive week, I decided to join the sea of people blogging about their thoughts and feelings and laying open their lives. What the hell, we're in the digital age, the time of big brother and days filled catching up with what people had for lunch or posting a ton of pictures of a sleeping cat (guilty as charged :-)), so why fool myself into thinking that anything is a sacred secret. Besides, I'm not a secretive person. As a natural wannabe writer, I tend to want to share easily what's in my head or my heart or on my plate or what I'm wearing or who's pissed me off.

So, here I am breaking my blogging virginity to make sense of my life and my struggles dealing with trying to get that family that comes so easily to everyone else around me. As many of those out there, I am blogging to self-medicate and be my own therapist (hopefully with the help of all of you who happen to read and take part in my blog). I am not new to writing, or to keeping a somewhat disjointed diary, neither am I new to self-medicating or therapy, but as mentioned, I am new to blogging. So in the light of this, I ask anyone who I have invited to read my blog and those who have stumbled upon my site and have decided to give it a go, to bear with me and accept that it is going to be rough around the edges until I get the hang of things.

For those friends who have been with me from the beginning of my IVF journey in 2013 and who have always been there with whistles, pom-poms, hugs or kisses, I thank you with all my heart. It is only because I have had you guys with me, that I am still (semi) sane and able to carry on.

I don't know what the structure of this blog will be, or if there will even be a structure. I have no plan, other than to share and communicate and invite others to do the same.

One thing, I would like everyone to take note of, is that I am going to be very much myself and how I feel and think at the time. If anyone (friends included), get offended by anything I say, please don't take it as a personal attack, as it won't be intended as such. Please accept me for who I am and how I am trying to deal with things, without judgement. Just because something might disagree with you in minor or even major areas of life, it doesn't mean that I don't value you as a person or friend or that I don't respect you for who you are or what you believe.

So, after that has been said, I welcome you to Where's My Stork- my (in)fertility trip of ups and downs in pursuit of my dream – to be mommy. I don't know where or how this story will end. Will I have the happy ending baby in my arms? Or will I have a happy ending with no baby? Either way, I plan to have a happy ending. I am tired of wasting life on being unhappy because of this disease called infertility (and it is a disease, believe you me). Whatever happens, and whichever direction this story takes, I plan to make sure it has a happy ending, somehow.

Love to all,
Bianca

Diary Entry 2
Walking on Sunshine
Published by Bianca on 7 April 2015

Summer in the UK seems to be here with a sudden burst. It's amazing the difference a few days can make. Last week I was still clutching at a thick jacket hiding from the wind and now I sit here in the summeriest (yes I made this word up) of summeriest clothes :-).

Unfortunately, I have somewhat wasted this good weather of the Easter weekend – which is something one should not do in the UK as one never knows whether the sun will be in town the following day or not. So why then have I wasted the good weather? I spent 4 days – yes 4 full days – lying on my bed watching episodes of *Prison Break*.

I didn't plan on having a long weekend of marathon TV watching. It just kind of happened that way due to the bloody hormones turning me into Little Miss Misery. My wonderful hubby tried everything he could – when I say everything, I mean everything from waiting on me hand and foot, to extra cuddles (that's a rarity for his Northern English blood) and even pulling funny faces – see the desperation there?! After my sad puppy eyes vomited out tears for no reason I could think of (bloody hormones), he finally decided to give up and join me in my misery on the bed. And there went the long weekend. Not a thing was accomplished. Not one single thing.

Now the guilt has set in. I look back at that crying little misery and I shake my head in disbelief. Why do I give in to ridiculous feelings which come from nowhere and are going nowhere? Why can't I just see them for what they are (stupid hormonal medication!), shrug it off and get along with life? So now I sit here on Tuesday feeling awful for the last 4 days and a silly cycle of more misery creeps in. Welcome to IVF. Welcome to hormonal treatments. Welcome to my current miserable life.

On the physical side, I think my new stomach tabs might be helping my ulcer – it is feeling much better than it has felt in a while, so fingers crossed my stomach lining is on the way to a proper recovery. My body has a medicated bloat and my skin is unrecognisable – hundreds of red blotches all over my face, neck and arms. It's like I've been invaded by a party load of adolescents hitting puberty! I feel disgusting. I feel the call of a dark corner where the world can't see me.

Outside the sun shines brightly. Bleh!

Diary Entry 3
Procrastination, Stuck in a Rut and Idle Hands making Devil's Work
Published by Bianca on 13 April 2015

This week started off with my husband annoying the crap out of me and no matter how much he tried to be nice or beg me to be nice, I just wasn't having any of it. This led to an argument, him storming out of the house and me planning to blog every angry detail about him in proper swanky words - my frustrations and details about the argument. Well, a few minutes later he called to apologise for being a dick and we made up and said 'I love yous'.

Yes, he was a dick who needed to apologise but so was I.

As mentioned in my previous entry, last week we wrote off Easter weekend - me through pure misery and my hubby after complete failure to lift me up. Tuesday was a work day. Wednesday to Friday was filled with clinic appointments, so none of these could be devoted fully to work or doing anything constructive. There's something about clinic days that injects both me and hubs with an overload of laziness juice. We always tend to get home from the clinic appointments and amble over to the lazy boy chairs in the lounge, only stopping in the kitchen on the way for crisps, nuts and chocolates to stuff our faces with as we binge watch a series on Netflix.

It has suddenly dawned on me that this pure laziness is not good for a healthy relationship with myself, my husband, my family, friends or with life. It is just a massive breeding ground for arguments and bitterness! Ya think? Well done me for finally realising the obvious!

It's been easy to get stuck in a rut. It crept up on us. A lazy day here and one there and next minute you we've had 4 consecutive days of nothing constructive which has become weeks, months and in danger of being years of numbness. I don't want to blink and my life is over without me having enjoyed it. My life and subsequently my husband's life at this moment is just living from cycle to cycle. The time in between cycles becomes dead time – merely the excruciating ticking of the clock to pass another 24 hours. Each episode takes away an hour of dead time and brings us a little closer to the next IVF cycle, the start of the next lot of meds, or egg retrieval, or embryo transfer, or pregnancy test day and hopefully our ultimate result - that little miracle in our arms. After a day's worth of episodes, we have gotten rid of at least 8 hours of dead time.

Why has this become our life? Well, going through these fertility challenges also brings our favourite words of *when* and *if*. Such as, '*When I'm off the meds, I will accept a party invitation* '. The meds are a great excuse for turning down anything we might consider to be fun, because oh no, how could we possibly have fun while on this hormonal / emotional roller coaster from hell?! And '*If we are pregnant then we will do up the spare room in the house, paint and make it pretty*' (as if we don't deserve pretty things unless we can give birth to one) and '*If this cycle fails, then I will find a new hobby, like drawing or writing, or making clothes.*' Why should starting a new hobby be dependent on feeling like a miserable failure? Procrastination! Stuck in a miserable rut.

But…I have decided that NOW is the time to find the joy and happiness, the fun and the laughter in life –things that will enrich my mind, warm my heart and make my soul sing. Now!!!! I don't want to wish my time away anymore. I don't want to have dead time or mindless blank spaces of nothingness in between cycles or events. I want to make the most of each hour of each day. NOW.

So, this week, and the week after that and after that, Vinny and I will get up and live life not just pass time!!

Diary Entry 4
Meant to be or not meant to be – No such thing
Published by Bianca on 22 April 2015

I have been harbouring a secret and I was waiting to report good or bad news.

Sadly, it's not the news I wanted to share.

In Feb of this year, the hubby and I spent our honeymoon doing IVF in Brno, Czech Republic – that was our 5th overall round of IVF and our first using donor eggs. We transferred two great embryos, but our babies were no shows. We had a good frozen embryo to transfer as back-up.

A few weeks ago, on Wednesday 8th of April, we packed a little bag each and drove again to London Stansted Airport to catch a flight to Brno, Czech Republic. I was already off work for 2 weeks as the college, where I teach closed for Easter, so I took an extra week leave after that to ensure a complete stress-free wait between transfer and testing day. That's also the reason why we didn't tell too many people that we were going. While it is common knowledge that I like to share and don't hold too many secrets, sometimes I feel a bit weighed down by everyone's anticipation of the next cycle working. Don't get me wrong, I am very happy that my support circle says prayers, crosses fingers, or does a little dance to the skies asking for my miracle (you know how much I value all of you), but at each failure, I feel like I have disappointed everybody and I feel like more of a failure. Sometimes too much sharing can get too much and feel heavy.

Anyway, this time we went to Brno for 3 days/2 nights rather than 7. It felt like such a drag now that we were there again within such a short time. This time wasn't as exciting. We had seen the sights, experienced all the new things and we had lost some of that hope we had packed into our suitcases previously.

Our doctor had no explanation for what could have gone wrong. They had been perfect top-grade embryos. All he could suggest was a steroid shot and daily blood thinning injections (Fraxiparine) – that was *fun*! I also had 2 more intralipid infusions.

3 Days later we came home and set about being as happy and stress free as possible. I relaxed for a few days doing nothing. Then I cleaned the house here and there and spent a lot of my time writing. Vinny and I spent good time together and laughed and dared to think about the embryo inside as 'our baby'. I had some unusual twinges and sharp stabbing cramps every now and then. I was extra thirsty. I peed a hell of a lot more than usual – getting up sometimes twice in the night. I didn't sleep too well. My breasts seemed to be changing shape. All good signs! I was happy. We were happy and yesterday morning when I woke up (again) for a pee at 3 am I couldn't wait to see those double pink lines.

I waited and waited and waited some more. This couldn't be happening again?! What the f*&$k!!!!!???!!!?????? Vinny couldn't believe it either. He urged me to check the test again and again, which I did. Still that one mocking line. It's strange, I had felt so different this time. The other times I have felt toward the end that it didn't work, as I got pms, was moody and had that period bloat with the spotty period skin – this time nada. Nothing like that. I stopped all meds yesterday and still don't feel like my period is coming. I keep having these sneaky thoughts that the test is faulty. But I know that's just creating emotional pain and could drive me crazy when I should just accept it and move on. Bloody progesterone!!!! The clinics do warn and I can attest to it, that the progesterone mimics pregnancy symptoms so one cannot rely on the 'feelings' – only on a positive test.

Then Vinny said to me, 'It's just not meant to be'.

I hate those words! I refuse to accept that things are either meant to be or not meant to be. If I must believe that, then I will always feel like a second-grade women or person even. Always ask questions like 'Why me?' If I accept that things are either meant to be or not meant to be, then tell *me why is the heroin addict meant to be pregnant injecting right through her pregnancy, while I try to keep myself as healthy as I can, but* **me** *falling pregnant is not meant to be? How is it meant to be for a baby to be born into an abusive household, while it's not meant to be for us who will love a baby with absolutely everything we've got? Why is it meant to be that some families have 8 children that they can't look after properly when we can't even get one?* NO!!!! If I must believe that my life is presupposed, then no matter what I do or don't do won't make an inch of difference and I will never be happy, so I refuse to believe that!!!

Life is both cruel and beautiful. Life happens to the best of people and the worst of people. Good things happen to both good and bad people and bad things happen to both good and bad people. Life doesn't have exceptions or favourites. Who am I to ask, 'Why me?' *The question should be 'Why not me?'* Why should it be someone else instead of me? Life itself has so many questions and we can ask and ask until the cows come home and never have a satisfactory answer. So, maybe we should just stop asking and keep doing the best we can with what we have. My life is what I make it, not what it is or isn't meant to be. Sometimes things work out the way I want them to and sometimes they don't. When they don't, I will keep trying my best to make it the way I want it. If I can't, then I hope that I will be able to enjoy the other opportunities that life offers.

"On some dimension or other, every event in life can be causing only one of two things: either it is good for you, or it is bringing up what you need to look at in order to create good for you."
Evolution is win-win…life is self-correcting."
— Deepak Chopra, *The Book of Secrets: Unlocking the Hidden Dimensions of Your Life*

Extra note…I follow a wonderful Buddhist Monk, called Ajahn Brahm. After writing this post, I realised that one of his latest talks is on this very subject and listening to it, has inspired me even more. Give yourself an hour from your day to relax, hop onto YouTube and listen to this awesome man for a little soul nourishment – you will not be disappointed!

Diary Entry 5
It's ok to be indulgent – just know when to stop
Published by Bianca on 28 April 2015

After last week's downer of a moment, this week was one of indulgence. Unfortunately, when it came to food, it was more like extreme over-indulgence – especially of the chocolate kind!!! I didn't think I would ever actually get sick from chocolate. But Saturday proved me wrong. After shovelling three quarters of a bottle of rich chocolate spread into my drooling mouth with a teaspoon, I didn't feel too good.

It didn't end there! Sunday night, my hubby decided to make his famously rich extra chocolatey chocolate chip giant cookies!!!!!!!! *How could I not cram 3 or 4 of those into my mouth fresh from the oven and then again for breakfast and another 2 or 3 after dinner on Monday night???!!!!?*

Back to Saturday…the chocolate spread might not have been the only contributing factor to my date with the toilet bowl, it could also have been the glass and a half of Moet and Chandon I had that didn't blend too well with the spread. I was tired of looking at the opened bottle of champagne every time I opened the fridge (left over from our wedding in Feb). Sure, it had gone flat weeks ago, but mixed with orange juice to make a Mimosa it tasted like I had just opened the bottle – minus the fizz. I hadn't had a drink since I over did it (mmm…..I see a pattern forming here) on the day of my previous negative pee stick in March – the night out that pushed my already suffering stomach ulcer to bleeding point – so I was keen to give it a go. Also, I was celebrating a little personal victory…

Me, the queen of the low pain threshold tribe, braved Vicky's tattoo gun at Down the Rabbit Hole Tattoo Studio in Gloucester where I went to get my first ink!! It was a wedding present from my husband. I am over the moon that I was able to sit there for half an hour without feinting, crying, screaming or vomiting. I did it!! Nearly 40 years old and finally got my first tattoo. Whoo hoo!!!! Ok granted, it's a little one, but I never thought I would even be able to endure that. I love it to bits! And so does my hubby. Hence the little celebration (of our love and marriage enduring pain) with the chocolate spread and left over bubbly :-).

Got to get back to some kind of exercise now!!!!

Diary Entry 6
Don't Fight Just Dance
Published by Bianca on 04 May 2015

This week has had its ups and downs for me. It started off quite good but then as soon as my clinic instructed me to add a steroid (Prednisone in the US/ Predisolone in the UK) to my mix of drugs, my husband freaked out. So before I even started taking them, he was already jumping at everything I said or didn't say or did or didn't do. He has this annoying habit of *predicting* how I am going to react in any given circumstance that hasn't even happened yet. If I frown a few seconds longer than what he thinks I usually do, I'm succumbing to the steroids. If I don't smile quick enough for his judgement or respond instantaneously to something he has said, the (hormonal) bitch is back. Then he takes up the attacking position to strike before he is struck down, because to be in a position of defence is to be vulnerable.

I have to admit, *this is not fully his fault*. We are all a product of our experiences and my husband, being an ex-military man as well as an ex-boxer, is only doing what he has been trained to do. When engaged with the enemy on the battlefield, or punching it out in the ring, this thinking will save his life, or win him a coveted title – either way, it will give him the advantage over his opponent.

What he fails to realise, is that I am not the enemy, our home is not a battlefield and there is no reason to try and get any advantage over anything.

In the real world, **assumption is definitely the mother of all fuck-ups**. There is no way of knowing how someone is going to react to something – there's only assuming. In assuming, you end up creating the environment that you are trying to prevent by throwing the first punch.

My tips *(to myself)* for the week....

Don't assume

It's not their fault – love them anyway (It's not my fault – love me anyway)

Don't fight back, just blog

Music heals the soul. Put on an album you love – have a cry, have a scream, have a dance around your lounge/bedroom/office. Just get lost in the words, the voice, the beat, the melody, the vibrations. My favourites this week come from Sons of Anarchy.

Battleme –Difficult to pick just one top song, but if I had to choose one, I would say the very first one of theirs that I heard, which was a cover of a Neil Young song called *Hey, Hey My My* (Into the Black), but Battleme do it so hauntingly beautiful – every hair on my body rises. Other good ones are *Burn this Town, Deadman, Big Score* and *Time* (with the Forest Rangers).

The White Buffalo – Gorgeous, raspy voice oozes passion. My favourites are *House of the Rising Sun* (SOA cover with a twist), *Come Join the Murder* (with the Forest Rangers), *Wish it was True* and *Oh Darlin what have I done?*

Noah Gundersen – The song *David* made me think of my own demons to slay – you will know what I mean when you hear the song.

Jack Savoretti – *Soldier's Eyes* – sad and beautiful – definite goosebump material

Ed Sheeren – Need I say more? *Make it Rain*

Awolnation – *Burn it Down* – this song is for some serious sweaty jumping around and going mental for a few minutes (after all the tear jerkers). Just act like a complete fun-loving idiot! It feels so good afterward :-).

To conclude this week's entry, as you may have guessed from the added steroid story above, we are indeed planning another trip to Brno, Czech Republic for transfer of one embryo. More on this soon.

Have a good week everyone!

Diary Entry 7
Be Like the Lotus Flower
Published by Bianca on 13 May 2015

Most people I have come into contact with since last Saturday know that I have a new edition to my body – brand new boldly coloured ink! It's still a month to go until my big 40, but with another embryo transfer coming up, I hope to be pregnant by the time my 40th is here – which meant another visit to Vicky at Down the Rabbit Hole Tattoo Studio in Gloucester :-). I might add that this is only my *second* tattoo (my first being my wedding ring *2 weeks ago*), and because I don't like doing things in half measures, I opted to go for a large red Lotus Flower emerging through blue waters as its roots wrestle with the mud below the water - beautifully displayed from shoulder to elbow. I am absolutely in love with it!! I love the design, the colours, the symbolism and how it makes me feel to look at it.

I have felt an affinity with the Lotus Flower for a long time now and this, dear friends, is why…

The Lotus Flower has been a sacred symbol across nations and religions. The life cycle of the Lotus Plant is a metaphor for human resolve. It is born in mud at the bottom of a pond, so its stalk needs to push through the mud and murky water to the surface where a radiant flower blooms as it faces the sun. Many ancient and modern cultures have used this plant to symbolise how a humble person should strive to rise above the gloomy thoughts, stresses and sadness of daily life to become a better and happier person in spite of one's origins or what one has had to face in life to get to the point of bloom.

The Confucian scholar Zhou Dunyi famously said, *'I love the lotus because while growing from mud, it is unstained.'*

Ancient Egypt – this flower was associated with *rebirth*, the *sun* and *creation* – as they believed it retracted into the water at night and emerged fresh and beautiful in the sun the next day.

Indian and Asian poetry – the image of the lotus is used to symbolise the *divine feminine*–the ideal female traits, as well as a metaphor for the female anatomy.

Hindus – beauty, *fertility*, prosperity, spirituality, and eternity

Buddhism – the mud represents humans who are born into a world of suffering, which is an inevitable part of human existence in one way or another but our effort to push ourselves through this suffering, makes us stronger and stronger so that we are eventually able to break free of the muddy water and become a beautiful, pure flower shining in the light of the sun. *The flower petals represent rebirth – a change of ideas, an acceptance of a situation or the dawn after our darkest of moments.*

The colours of the flower petals also have several meanings, and I tried to take this into consideration when choosing my flower. I decided on red, which represents the heart – love, compassion, passion and other qualities of the heart.

Every day when I look at my Red Lotus Flower on my arm, I will be reminded that I am *strong enough* to push through the thickest of difficulties and *nothing will stop my heart from blooming. I am stronger than my troubles. I am a beautiful, complete women who will rise and shine radiantly in the sun no matter how much mud threatens to suffocate my roots.*

We can all be like the Lotus Flower.

In other news:
Transfer of our PGD CGH tested embryo on Saturday! This time a fully donated embryo (eggs and sperm – failproof!)

Diary Entry 8
Will Seven Be Our Number?
Published by Bianca on 20 May 2015

As you know, we have just taken a 3rd **trip** to our clinic in the Czech Republic for our 7th **IVF transfer**. Call it bravery, call it stupid stubbornness, call it blind madness, call it whatever you like, but regardless, we still have this compulsion to carry on, steroids and all, as we desperately cling to every fibre of hope carried on Ryanair wings, that we will get our miracle baby.

So, Thursday night we landed in Bratislava with our overnight bags and checked into the Hilton for some spoiling. Having a husband that stays in the Hilton regularly on business trips has its advantage, as we were given a luxury suite, plus a fabulous breakfast buffet spread.

After a short tour of Bratislava city and Bratislava Castle with its views far into Austria (although not quite that far on our grey and cloudy day), we caught the train to Brno (1.5-hour journey). This time we stayed at the luxurious Barcelo Hotel. I had a 90-minute Thai massage and Vinny appreciated the gym, sauna and jet showers, before a silver service ala carte dinner. We also enjoyed a great breakfast spread, cheap cocktails and very late check-out. All round, the hubby and I had an absolute ball – our only regret – that we didn't arrange to stay longer and sit lazily in the sun sipping on Pivo at one of the many street cafes. Quite a different feeling to our previous trip a month before, where we ate snacks for dinner in our (basic) hotel room and waited at the airport for 6 hours to check in simply because we had nowhere to go and it was far too cold to sit outside!

Saturday was transfer day! We saw a different doctor who decided that it was time we took the 'less is more' approach – *no more* intralipid infusions, *no* steroid shot, *no more* daily blood thinning injections – only my daily oral steroid (which incidentally has given me what is termed a 'moon face' – yay), oestrogen and progesterone. Within half an hour, I was PUPO (pregnant until proven otherwise) with one PGD CHI tested donated embryo.

So as we wait to test and find out whether that perfect embryo has found an optimum place to attach and implant, and eventually become our baby, I've been wondering how to calm my restless spirit and keep a positive momentum going for 12 long (*long, long, long*) days. Then it suddenly flashed in my head like a slot machine ringing 'jackpot!' *The number SEVEN – 7 – the world's favourite and luckiest digit!*

From one end of an ancient piece of the world to another end of modern civilization, and across both western and eastern cultures and religions, *the number 7 has been a remarkable, special, magical number.*

In the *Christian Bible*, the number 7 is the number of completeness and perfection in both the physical and the spiritual, tied directly to God's creation. It is used 735 times, while the word sevenfold appears 6 times and seventh appears 119 times, making the total reference to the number 7 in the Bible 860 times.

Judaism claims the universe consists of 7 heavens, while 7 traditional blessings are said at a wedding and the bride circles her groom 7 times.

The *Hindus* believe there to be 7 higher worlds and 7 underworlds.

There are 7 Gods of Fortune in *Japanese Mythology*.

The newborn *Buddha* rose to his feet and took 7 steps.

The *Quran* also speaks about 7 heavens, while Muslim pilgrims to Mecca walk 7 times around the Kaaba (the building which is the centre of Islam's most sacred Mosque).

In *China*, the number 7 is considered lucky as the word sounds like the Chinese word for arise / life / birth.

Other references to the number seven:

The human body has 7 basic chakras.

There are 7 colours of the rainbow.

7 is the winning numbers in the slots.

David Beckham wore the number 7 for Manchester united. His daughter's middle name is Seven. (Incidentally, one of my own good friends named his son Seven and has the number 7 tattooed down his back from neck to tail.)

There are 7 wonders of the ancient world.

There are also 7 wonders of the modern world, which were decided by global ballot, the results of which were announced on the 7th day of 7th month 2007.

*** This is our 7th IVF transfer *** – See my point in this?

Now, I am by no means a religious person, or a great believer in things like tarot cards or numerology or magic numbers, which is quite an interesting statement in itself, because since this IVF journey, as most of us in the same fertility challenged position, I have grabbed onto any speck of possibility that magic does exist, by surrounding myself with a multitude of gem stones, carrying little angel figurines in my pocket, wearing the 'lucky' colour red, praying to every God's name I can think of and whatever else anyone has suggested over the last 2 years!

All that said, I am not that naive into thinking that this transfer is a sure thing now because of a number. It has a 50/50 chance like all the others (well the others had a 35 percent chance – the odds are better with this one as its PGD CHI tested using donated chromosomes from a 21 and 23-year-old!). But, if nothing else, at least believing in the Number Seven for 12 days will keep the hope alive!

And maybe, just maybe, our 7th transfer is the special one, where we will find our pot of gold, our miracle baby, at the end of the magical rainbow ;-

).

Bianca   xxx

Side Entry (Additional Notes)
Our IVF in BRNO, Czech Republic

Our **first** trip to Brno was exciting. We had just got married and we planned to use these 7 days away for IVF as a little honeymoon (not my first choice for a honeymoon but it was all we had to work with), visiting *Prague*, *Vienna* and *Bratislava* (none more than 3 hours way by train) plus explore the quaint town of Brno. We truly had a fantastic time! We flew an hour and a half from Stansted on Ryanair and were tucked into our apartment soon after. It was beautiful - modern minimalist chic. The apartment coordinator, Lucy, was very helpful and always on the other side of an email. It was a great find and if you're ever in Brno, look up Bishop's Apartments.

On our **second** trip was only for 2 nights so we tried the VV Hotel. It was great. Again, they had the modern chic look with plenty of space. It was pretty, comfortable and clean with a window that opens wide for fresh air. The view wasn't great – an old construction site and a strip club, but hey we weren't there for the view! Heating was good for the winter months. The continental breakfast overflowed with all sorts of goodies. Two free bottles of water in the room every day and water, juice and coffee/tea available free of charge throughout the day in the breakfast area. The staff spoke a little English and were friendly and accommodating. The TV channels were mostly in Czech, French and German with CNN & BBC News being the only English channels – we watched preloaded movies on a laptop. Overall, it was a good experience and we would stay there again.

For our **third** trip, we decided to do things a little differently. This time we flew from Birmingham to Bratislava (avoiding London helped cut down travel time to the airport). Thanks to the hubby being a Hilton Diamond Club member due to his many business trips over the last 2 years, we had a free night in an executive suite at the Double Tree Hilton with amazing free breakfast spread.

Our clinic appointment was on the Saturday, so we flew the Thursday night, spent the day in Bratislava exploring the town and castle and then caught a train (1.5 hours away and 10 Euros each one way) to Brno.

We went extra luxury this time and chose the hotel, Barcelo Brno Palace, where we indulged in pre-dinner happy hour cocktails (*they have yummy virgin cocktails too*), ala carte dinner, 90-minute Thai massage (me) and gym, sauna and jet shower (hubby). The hotel had an air of relaxation – perfect for transferring precious little embryos – from the comfy rooms, to the glass lifts, elegant lobby, delicious food and outstanding service. The price was great too – far less than you would pay for the same anywhere in the UK. We had a great time! A big bonus for us, was the late check-out – until 16.00 for only 15 Euros. After check-out we sat in the lobby playing cards over refreshments for about 2 hours and then leisurely caught our train back to Bratislava for our 22.30 flight. Oh and, the airport in Bratislava was much better than Brno – more choice in shops and restaurants!

Why did we go to Eastern Europe?

IVF in the UK can be free for 1 to 3 cycles depending on the post code you live in (plus some other factors such as age). Vinny and I are one of the lucky couples who live in a post code that offers 3 rounds of IVF paid for by the NHS (National Health Service). Round 4, which was our one little frozen embryo that we got from our second egg collection, we had to pay for ourselves (*still over £2,000 for transferring the embryo after paying £1000 for freezer storage*). That was *just* doable for us on already maxed-out credit cards, but any more treatments were not looking too good in the UK financially. To top that, we were told by local fertility specialists that the technology in Europe far exceeds that in the UK, resulting in higher success rates. **Really?! So, Europe was cheaper with more advanced technologically and higher success rates?! What were we waiting for???**

The main European centres for IVF are Spain, Greece and the Czech Republic. I let the fact that the time had come for *donor* eggs (according to our fertility specialist in the UK), decide where we were going. I am naturally fair-skinned and fair-haired, and I am half German with typical European features. Both my grandparents on my father's side were born in Czech - not only that, but they were both born in the very town where one of the top clinics are, *Brno*, so that adds a little meaning into the mix. The Czech Republic seemed the no-brainer choice for us.

About price…as an example, a fresh donor egg cycle at my original clinic in the UK is over £8,000, excluding medication which they estimate at around £400 give or take. A trip for the both of us to Czech including flights, accommodation, fresh donor egg cycle, medication and intralipid infusions (these alone are *from £172 right up to £700 per go depending on the clinic in the UK*), was roughly £4,000.00. And everything else like food, drink and transport is extremely cheap. We also spent less in Czech for weekly groceries than we do in the UK.

As it was our first time going to the Czech Republic, we decided that we would feel more confident going through a local coordinator. A great thing about using the coordinating company is that we could jump the egg donor waitlist, and a cycle from beginning to transfer could take as little as 6 weeks! We were happy to pay the £375 service charge for this alone.

Preparation

We filled in a stack of forms (as we have done everywhere hundreds of times!), now with added details on our preferred egg donor – looks, education and interests, then it was wait for my protocol and confirmation dates.

<u>My Protocol included</u>:

* *Birth control pills* for fresh donor egg cycle, to sync my cycle with the donor's cycle and be ready by our chosen date. These didn't agree with me, and by the 5th day I couldn't get out of bed from the nausea, vomiting and migraines. I was taken off them immediately and prescribed another type of synthetic progesterone hormone.

* *Intramuscular Injection* for my fresh donor cycle, administered in the butt muscle by a medical professional, to lower my oestrogen levels.

* *Oestrogen Pills* for both my fresh and frozen cycles, to thicken the lining of my uterus.

**Progesterone Pills* for both fresh and frozen cycles, to balance out the oestrogen and to turn my uterus into a favourable environment for the embryo(s).

* *Steroids* with both fresh and frozen cycles, to suppresses my immune system which could be trying to fight off the embryo(s) as a foreign object.

* *Intralipid infusions* for both fresh and frozen cycles, also to suppress my immune system.

* *Iron supplements* to combat anaemia – throughout IVF treatment.

* *Aspirin* to prevent blood clots.

* Folic Acid.

** *Trans-vaginal ultrasound scan* to measure the thickness of my endometrial lining. The oestrogen helps the lining to grow around 1 mm a day. A few days before egg collection, my lining was at 6.4 mm and optimal is 8 to 11.

For us as a couple: No more sex for the next 7 weeks.

For my hubby: No ejaculation 2 to 3 days before giving sperm on (donor's) egg collection day!

Treatment at Reprofit, Brno

Fresh Donor Egg Cycle (First Cycle in Brno)

* We had to be in Brno for at least 7 nights from one day before egg/sperm collection to one day after transfer.

* On egg / sperm collection, I had a quick scan to make sure that my lining was growing as thick as expected (*by that stage it had grown over 2 mm in two days, and was now 8.6 mm*), as well as my first intralipid infusion, which took around 90 min.

* We had a consultation with our assigned doctor and was told that our donor had produced 11 eggs, which was excellent! She was 25 years old, blonde, green eyes, 1.62 m tall, slim and had a bachelor's degree. She had a proven track record of 2 previous pregnancies from her donated eggs. Perfect!

* The next day we received the fertilization results – 9 of the eggs fertilized – great news!

* Two days later we had 3 excellent embryos, 3 good embryos and 2 that were just ok.

Fantastic news! So, we had a confirmed day 5 transfer.

* On transfer day, we had:

1 x hatching blastocyst – grade 1 (top quality)

1x expanded blastocyst – grade 1 (top quality)

1 x blastocyst – grade 2

1 x early blastocyst – possibly degenerating

1 x compact morula with cavitation – no good

1x 10 cell embryo – no good

NOTE: Short explanations of these terms can be found on the word list at the end of this book.

* We also got the results of my husband's semen analysis which was done on collection day:

Normal Morphology (%) – 1 (him) and 4 (lowest limit) – OH DEAR!!??!

Semen Analysis Results – <u>Teratozoospermia</u> – what the f*$£k!!!???!! – Turns out, this is a type of male infertility – when the sperm is an abnormal shape and therefore cannot fertilize the egg on its own. Severe Teratozoospermia is less than 5%! So, it seems that my dear husband has worse than a severe case. Apparently, the chances of conceiving naturally are next to zero but egg fertilization is still possible with ICSI (where the sperm is injected into the egg rather than let it try and reach the egg naturally).

With all 3 fresh IVF cycles at Oxford Fertility Clinic, we always had the ICSI backup, but had never needed it, which means that his sperm has not always been like this but has deteriorated at an alarming rate - within 5 months!!! Scary stuff!

* We transferred both grade 1 embryos and had one embryo to freeze.
* Transfer was on a semi-full bladder and took 5 min. We could see the embryos on the big screen and the placement of them in my uterus on the monitor! After they were transferred, I lay on the bed for a further 15 min to allow them to settle and then had a second intralipid infusion.

The main instructions for the next two weeks:
1) no bed rest – I needed to move to prevent blood slowing down and

possible clots

2) no heavy lifting or vigorous exercise - to prevent muscles from pulling or cramping

3) no baths, swimming or immersing in water - to prevent any possible infections

4) no sex for at least the next 5 days – also to prevent infections (as if we hadn't been abstinent for the last 6 weeks!!!)

Result of our first fresh donor egg cycle: FAIL! NOT PREGANT.

Result of our frozen egg donor transfer: FAIL! NOT PREGNANT.

Result of our fully donated (and genetically tested) EMBRYO: FAIL! NOT PREGNANT.

Diary Entry 9
Keeping The Dream Alive
Published by Bianca on 31 May 2015

If you have been following my blog regularly, then you might already know that our 7th IVF cycle fail. I have been grieving, gathering my strength, working on picking myself up again and brainstorming our next move, which so far changes several times a day.

One thing we are sure of, is that there **will be** a next move, the details of which I will go into at a later stage when we have more of a fixed direction ourselves. For now, I am *"meditating"* on my favourite story, *Alice in Wonderland*. So this week, I will leave you with a few of the best quotes from the story, and I challenge you to put aside your adult/logical brain and open up the mind of the child within you and keep dreaming about and believing in what you want in life, because that is what I will be doing…

Have a good week everyone.

"Sometimes I believe as many as 6 impossible things before breakfast."

"You, he said, are a terribly real thing in a terribly false world, and that I believe is why you are in so much pain."

"I knew who I was this morning but I've changed a few times since then."

"The mad hatter — have I gone mad?
Alice — I'm afraid so. you're entirely bonkers but I tell you a secret, all the best people are."

Bianca Xxx

Diary Entry 10
Don't Let Those Hormones Beat You!
Published by Bianca on 7 June, 2015

This last week I have been trying to find my feet in the real world once again after being on Planet PUPO (*pregnant until proven otherwise*) and then slammed into the world of 'Proven Otherwise!' with my negative test.

Now for those who don't know, dealing with this shift from excitement, to hope, to disbelief and disappointment, not only has its intellectual difficulties as the brain tries to grasp what the hell just happened (again!), but the immediate shift from living in a depressing bubble of chemicals a.k.a. hormonal and steroidal medication, back to an equally depressing chemical nakedness, is physically punishing, which in turn pushes the full spectrum of emotions to feverish delirium.

This time really hit me harder than I expected. Perhaps it was the steroids, which amplified all the usual effects, coupled with the haunting thought that if properly tested 'perfect' donated embryos failed to implant, it must be a confirmation that my womb has been the rubbishing culprit all along. That made me extra sad, which turned me into a bad-tempered miserable blubbering discombobulated mass of tears and anger for my lucky husband to enjoy!

Every time I snapped at the tiniest of inconveniences, or just didn't *feel* like smiling, or acted petulantly, I would blame it on the hormones. Then one day as I sweated away doing my exercises on the Xbox (by the way, a wonderful form of meditation and therapy!), it occurred to me that human beings are so skilled at blaming everything on something. Blame. Blame. Blame. And for those of us doing IVF, it becomes a *dirty* habit to blame every bad feeling, action and reaction on IVF and those *bloody* hormones to the point of taking no responsibility for ourselves. In psychology, they call this victim mentality.

Don't get me wrong, I am not saying all those hormones, other medication, failed cycles and everything else that goes along with IVF and trying to conceive are not responsible for the way I feel. They most certainly are! *However*, **I am responsible for what I do with those feelings. I have a choice. I can choose to be eaten up and spat out by my own sadness and fury or I can choose to rise above it.**

So, in continuing with my meditation while exercising, my next thought was about my husband going away soon for 3 weeks of work. What if we never saw each other again? Morbid thought I know, but life has no guarantees, and anything could happen to either one of us before he arrives back home. What kind of last memories together would I want to create? Would those tiny inconveniences that irritated me really be important at all? Would I really want his last image of me to be of red eyes, and my last words to be cutting and icy? Would I really want to let hormones and a failed IVF cycle ruin our precious time together if I knew I would never see him again? NO!

So then, why was I letting it? Why was I letting this setback pump negativity into moments that should be filled with smiles, laughter and love?

I love my husband more than anything in this world. He is my soul mate. I love him more than any anger and more than my sadness. The love I have within me is stronger than any effects of hormones, or steroids or failed IVF cycles and I refuse to allow the difficulties of this fertility journey to become bigger than that love and to rob us of the happiness we have right now. Whether we have a baby tomorrow or never, I am still incredibly blessed to have so much love in my life and I won't wait until tomorrow to show him how grateful and happy I am for having him. Today and every day *will* have love and laughter despite the bloody hormones!

Diary Entry 11
I'll get by with a little help from my friends
Published by Bianca on 17 June 2015

Most of you will know that last week was my 40th birthday, but many of you won't know that I spent most of my day crying. No…that's putting it too mildly. I spent most of my day *sobbing* – with whiny sounds and everything. My husband always says that I go supersonic when I cry (useful if I lived with a pod of dolphins or whales, but neither he nor my cats are ever impressed).

Birthdays have often been a struggle for me, especially the last 10 years with every childless year that goes by *highlighting my use-by date for motherhood.* Before the day came around, I decided that this time I was going to have a good day regardless. *And what do you know?* No word of a lie, 2 minutes past midnight, a dense cloud of doom descended over me and the first salty tear trickled into my mouth. I can't say whether I subliminally sabotaged my day or whether it was just bad luck and bad timing after all the weight and stresses of this fertility journey. It was probably a mix of so many factors – age, constant cycle failures, on again/off again meds, a realization that we have spent 90 % of the past two years solely centred around IVF and have missed out on so much of life with no return for our

44

investment yet (if ever) and the start of the US portion of my husband's work, meaning that we will hardly see each other over the next 3 to 6 months (*a sad and lonely thought for someone going through IVF – your partner becomes more of a partner than ever on this journey – he is my rock and my lifeline*).

With every possible negative thought piling one on top of the other, I became so tired and worn out, suddenly drained of all hope, ready to give it all up. A good friend of mine had made plans to take me out for celebrations, but I knew that forcing fun was going to be futile – I was beyond miserable. My face was not going to entertain any sort of smile. So, I cancelled a party evening in favour of an evening in bed with a defrosted Black Forest Gateaux, a bottle of bubbly chilling in the fridge and back to back episodes of Nashville.

Two glasses in, I was still filling up storm drains with my not so attractive puffy peepers. Desperate times called for desperate measures and it was time for back-up.

Enter my fellow IVF warriors from my online support group.

About 20 incredible women came to my immediate rescue with oceans of encouragement and love. With every message, my strength grew, as did my appreciation, admiration and wonder until all that negative stuff couldn't stand to stay around anymore. What made this extra special for me, was not only that these ladies haven't known me for that long, or that we haven't actually met in person, but that each and every one of them has their own suitcases packed full of tears, struggles, heartache and fears caused by this horrible fertility situation we have found ourselves in. Yet, despite that, these fierce, determined, brave, loving, amazing warrior women put down their own heavy weight for a while, came together and pulled from their core, the strength and encouragement that someone else needed to get back in the fight.

With their help, I decided to embrace and celebrate these 40 years of mine. Just because I am on a different path to the one I thought I would be on by the time I reached 40, just because I don't yet have children and the family of my dreams, just because I am fighting this bitter disease, does **NOT** make me any less of a person or woman, or mean that I have nothing to celebrate. ***I have MANY accomplishments to be proud of and celebrate.*** I love the way one of the ladies put it…

"it's good to recognise another year of increased wisdom and knowledge and honour the survivor within."

But in addition, I will say that I am much more than a survivor. I am a warrior. I am a superhero in my own story. I am proud of the person that I have become on my journey to 40!

Aesop said, *"No act of kindness, no matter how small is ever wasted."*

Words, a virtual hug or kiss, a prayer at home, a relevant article, a beautiful picture, a joke to make me giggle, any form of reaching out to me – it's all appreciated more than you know.

I raise my glass of bubbly to toast and say thank you to everyone near and far, old friends and new friends, who have been there for me and helped me get this far. I celebrate you!

Bianca xxx

p.s. After applying tea bags and iced spoons to the big lumps where my eyes usually are, my lovely friend collected me the following night for a party and let me tell you anything negative still left inside was sweated out on the dance floor! It was a great night!

p.p.s. Last night I officially became a British Citizen. 6.5 Years ago, I decided to change my life forever. I got on a plane from South Africa with my 20kg suitcase and landed in London alone, not knowing where I would work or live or how I would survive. Here I am living a wonderful life with my amazing soul mate, my 2 beautiful cats, fantastic friends, an added degree and teaching qualification and loads, loads more! Not that I didn't have help along the way, but I feel that I can be damn proud of myself.

p.p.p.s. I decided to make myself a **Feel Good** playlist…check it out below and have a mad dance around when you're in need of a boost…

*My theme song for this post in honour of all of you is **I'll be there for you (The Rembrandts)**. One of my all-time favourite songs from one of my all-time favourite sitcoms!

"…It's like you're always stuck in second gear. And when it hasn't been your day. Your week. Your month. Or even your year, but I'll be there for you. No-one could ever know me. No-one could ever see me. Seems you're the only one who knows. What it's like to be me. Someone to face the day with. Make it through all the rest with. Someone that I'll always laugh with. Even at my worst I'm best with you…"

*Waka Waka (Shakira) – This was the official World Cup Football 2010 song. I'm a little biased on this one as the World Cup was in South Africa that year and the song has an African vibe to it. I can't help but feel good and happy to be a strong South African when this song comes on!

"...You're a good soldier. Choosing your battles. Pick yourself up. And dust yourself off. Get back in the saddle. When you fall get up...If you fall get up..."

*It's Amazing (Aerosmith) – Such a beautiful song that always lifts my spirit.

"...There were times in my life. When I was going insane. Tryin' to walk through the pain...
...It's amazing. With the blink of an eye. You finally see the light...When the moment arrives that you know you'll be alright..."

*Tubthumping (Chumbawamba) – an old one but who doesn't like this get up and go song?! Incidentally another Football World Cup song (1998).

"...I get knocked down but I get up again, you're never gonna keep me down. He sings the songs that remind him of the good times. He sings the songs that remind him of the better times..."

*Roar (Katy Perry) – with songs such as these which are written about relationships or something similar, I always imagine the villain to be infertility and I sing out loud with the aim of overcoming these struggles.

"... I got the eye of the tiger, the fire...Cause I'm a champion and you're gonna hear me roar..."

*Bad Day (Daniel Powter) – another classic from way back then. But oh oh oh, such a good one! Love this song and somehow it always makes me smile and puts me in such a good mood. I can't help bellowing it out whenever I hear it (although that's not a good thing as singing is soo not one of my talents!)

"…You had a bad day…You sing a sad song just to turn it around…You work at a smile and go for a ride…"

*We are the Champions (Queen) – Iconic winners' song!

"…We are the champions my friend, And we'll keep on fighting till the end…"

*Ain't no mountain high enough (Marvin Gaye & Tammi Terrell) – I am pretty sure all my fellow fertility warriors can relate to this song – there is no mountain high enough to climb if it means getting our family! On the other hand, it's also the essence of a supporting friend.

"…Ain't no river wide enough. To keep me from getting to you…"

*Survival (Muse) – A powerful force behind powerful words to ignite the winning fire within!

"…And I'll light the fuse. And I'll never lose. And I choose to survive. Whatever it takes…I'm gonna win…"

*Won't back down (Tom Petty and the Heartbreakers) – smooth listening with strong words that make give me encouragement.

"…Well, I know what's right, I got just one life. In a world that keeps on pushin' me around. But I'll stand my ground. And I won't back down…"

*Lean on Me (Bill Withers) – Speaks for itself. This is for all my fellow fertility warriors!

"…Lean on me. When you're not strong. And I'll be your friend. I'll help you carry on…"

*Never Surrender (Corey Heart) – Truth is I have never heard of this artist or this song before, but the words are just so apt that I had to put it in. Never surrender (to your demons)!

"Just a little more time is all we're asking for. Cause just va little more time can open closing doors. Just a little uncertainty can bring you down. And nobody wants to know you now…So if you're lost and on your own. You can never surrender. And if your path won't lead you home. You can never surrender. And when the night is cold and dark. You can see, you can see light. Cause no one can take away your right. To fight and never surrender…"

*Anything by AC/DC – one of the best bands in the world EVER! EVER!! *Who can sit still and be miserable when they come on the radio??!!?* I just want to run and jump around and go completely mental (in a good way of course!).

Diary Entry 12
Viva Espana!
Published by Bianca on 02 July 2015

Hola Amigos!

As you may have guessed, Vinny and I have just returned from a few days of sun, sea, swimming and Spanish speaking. Well, I had all good intentions of practicing my Spanish but once there I suddenly had a mouth full of marshmallows and could only mumble some strange sounds (despite my 6-week Spanish course just finished!). Next time I will be bolder!

Barcelona – what a great city! It has an energy that gently massages the senses (*except on garbage day, that's more of a direct assault on the nose, but we can overlook that for now*) and puts one in a dreamy trance - almost like walking in the air between clouds of puffy cotton wool.
The people are fantastic – full of life and sparkle with smiles to light up a 4th of July night sky.
Our hotel, the Hilton Diagonal Mar, wasn't too bad either. Poolside on the roof was awesome with live DJ playing chilled Miami beats while a Meet & Greet hostess escorted us to our extra cushioned sun loungers. She

magically appeared again at our sides like a glowing angel, when we merely glanced at the cocktail menu. My husband now lives in fear that I could get used to that kind of lifestyle. I remind him of his favourite mantra, *'happy wife, happy life'*. He smiles nervously.

But let me put all that aside and focus on the real reason we took this trip – our next dive into the Sea of (Fertility) Hope. On Monday we met with our new doctor and coordinator at IVI International. We had a frank discussion about our history, our expectations, our options, their suggestions and modus operandi. After discussing our history, the first thing the doc wanted to know was whether I had had a hysteroscopy. After a missed miscarriage on our first cycle and 6 subsequent implantation failures, she confirmed the truth of my own thoughts – that a hysteroscopy should have been an obvious procedure way back when…!!! **Finally, we feel like we are getting somewhere** – a doctor that is taking the initiative and giving us proper direction instead of leaving us to tread water and just clock up the cycles with a tweak of the meds!!

So, this is where we're at right now…

Initial Consultation

Bianca:

A shipload of bloods taken (Rubella, Sodium, Potassium, Iron, Gluten, GMTHFR mutation, full blood count and many others centred around implantation failure which I can't even pronounce…)

Initial scan and mock embryo transfer

Complete egg donor specification form (the clinic stressed that it would be difficult to find someone with my exact specifications – blonde hair and green eyes (it's Spain after all, you know that beautiful olive skin we all want!) – but at this stage we are beyond that. Besides, I've seen loads of children that don't look anything like their biological parents!

Vinny:

Half a shipload of bloods taken

Sperm given for the following tests:

Spermiogram (initial and general sperm test for volume, density and motility)

FISH (diagnosis of chromosomal anomalies in sperm cells)

TDG-D 549 + Karyotype (Genetic matching with egg donor to prevent genetic mutations) – takes 5 weeks for results

If the FISH comes back normal – nothing more will need to be done with Vinny's sperm.
If the FISH comes back with abnormalities – our embryos will be sent for PGD testing (4-week timeframe)

2 July 2015
Start birth control pills in order to manipulate my cycle to prepare for a procedure called **ERA** (test to pinpoint the day in a woman's cycle when

there is the best chance an embryo will successfully implant, which is not necessarily the same for every woman).

7 August 2015
ERA Test & Hysteroscopy (possibly a 3-day trip to Barcelona)

Mid September
Estimated date when donor begins medication

Mid October
Estimated date of embryo transfer

As you can see, all this is going to take some time and most of our plans for this year must be put on hold for now. Two years ago, I started my meds for my first IVF cycle on 11 July – what two years it has been, full of highs and lows, dreams and disappointments. Hopefully we won't need another two years. But we have tried the quick back to back cycles from December to May and 7 months later we are still 'at the beginning', so this time *we would rather do it right than quick.*

In the meanwhile, I am going to finesse these next 3 months. I'm not going to simply wait for time to go by and miss out on life. I have big plans to take control of myself rather than trying to control the uncontrollable. With the help of an awesome lady from my online support group, I am going to get out from under the thumb of infertility and the hold it has on me and put myself back into that thing called life!

I'm so excited about everything happening over the next few months and beyond! The next leg of my IVF journey is going to be an adventure, not a prison sentence!

Love & Hugs

B xxx

Diary Entry 13
Cheese with that whine?
Published by Bianca on 19 July 2015

As I start to write this, I have just woken up from a long sleep in the middle of the day with one cat stretched out at my side and another at my feet.

Bliss...

I wish I could stay like this for another few days – being a cat with my cats. My little fur babies, with their little marshmallow paws crossed over little fluffy bellies, always manage to draw out a smile from somewhere inside no matter how much I don't want to smile.
But this isn't a blog about cats, so let me move on...

Be warned. Brace yourselves. In fact, literally go and get a glass or bottle of wine because this post is all about me bitching! I'm sorry, but I've got to get it out. I've got to shovel it to throw it away and move on to the new week empty of all this rubbish. Next week's blog update will be back to sunshine and smiles from me.

For now though, take a deep breath and read on....or just stop reading now and go do something more interesting, I won't be offended. Either way, I need to write this today for myself!

As you know from my last post, Vin and I went to our first meeting with a new, highly recommended (and highly expensive) clinic in Barcelona. IVI Fertility has been promoted widely by the media in the UK and is the first choice for many UK clinics when it comes to egg donation and advanced technology. Yes, our initial consultation was constructive and encouraging. All the staff members were efficient. We had a myriad of tests done that we have never been offered before – all the standard plus more advanced genetic blood and semen tests. We made an appointment to go back for the ERA test and a hysteroscopy on the 7th of August. We paid a good chunk of Euros and went home full of sparkle, feeling lucky to have found IVI Fertility.

That feeling didn't last long.

*A day after arriving back home, we were told that we had been undercharged!

*We were also told that we should hold off booking our flights and accommodation for my hysteroscopy and ERA 7th August, even though the appointment had been made already made while we had been at the clinic.

*Three days later I was chasing a prescription for pills I needed to take within 5 days. I was finally emailed the prescription on the Friday and Monday was the latest I could start the pills. As all the big international clinics know, trying to get any medication in the UK while being treated abroad is virtually impossible. Pharmacies that are prepared to have a UK doctor rewrite the prescriptions are few and are usually only in London – 2.5 hours away and would therefore need a courier to get to me. I would never make it there before closing.

*Then my coordinator went on 4 days leave without telling me. I found out on her 'out of office' message when I emailed her a 5th time asking for confirmation of the 7th of August booking and for our test results. A week later (Thursday) I emailed her again, on the day her 'out of office' claimed she would be back. No reply. Next morning, I received an email from her telling me that she was no longer going to be my coordinator but that I should contact someone else and *by the way* the clinic could not perform my procedures on 7th August as the last operations for the summer were being done end of July.

*In fury, I emailed the new coordinator immediately, gave it a few hours and then phoned only to be told on the phone that the new coordinator chooses not to speak to me until she has become familiar with my file, and that could take a few days. I frantically searched their website for alternative telephone numbers and contact people to speak to.

That's when I found a long list of bad reviews from their patients. On their own website!

These ranged from:

*Very slow to practically no communication from the coordinators
*People told they haven't paid enough
*Getting patient test results mixed up

*Incorrect medicine prescribed

*Incorrect protocols

*Cold and uncaring

*Promises of finding a donor within 6 weeks and it took 6 months

*No donor eggs available on the day of transfer

*Forgetting to tell a patient when her transfer day was, and the cherry on top

*Got someone's sperm mixed up and then told the woman that if she is pregnant then she must wait for the baby to be born and do a DNA test to make sure that the sperm was her husband's!!!!

Fucking crazy. All these complaints were by different people and most of the complaints were the same things over and over. After I confronted the clinic about these reviews, they have subsequently taken them down and converted this patient forum to Spanish only! Quite a sly move. However, on the day I discovered them, I copied and pasted most of them to an email to Vin, so still have them as evidence.

As you might imagine, I was a complete mess after this! I was crying in that way that children cry when they can't get a breath. That like whooping cough kind of sound, you know? I couldn't believe this was happening to us. We were back to the beginning with no idea of where we should go from here.

And then a few hours later, out of the blue, in the afternoon of the same day that we were told that we couldn't have our procedures on the 7th of August, I received an email from the new coordinator saying that she was delighted to confirm that we can now have those procedures done as originally planned. *What?!?!* To this email, she had attached a treatment plan for the ERA test. *Treatment plan?* I had been given a prescription for one lot of pills a week before and not been told that I needed anything else. This plan included an injection to be administered by a nurse or doctor on Wednesday. This was Friday afternoon and I did not even have the prescription yet, let alone the medicine in order to make...no... beg my GP for an appointment! To top it all, we were going to Germany for the weekend and only back on Tuesday! **This was crazy. I was crazy – crazy mad, angry, furious!!**

Nothing more could be done over the weekend, but Monday morning they received a piece of Vinny's mind. It was time for the big guns – Vinny's! No more Mr Nice Guy. So, a torrent of emails went back and forth. In between these we received instructions for the hysteroscopy, including a list of meds (*again with no prescription*) and were told that I needed to do an ECG within the next two weeks and send them the results. What?! *Why would I need an ECG?* I have been under anaesthetic 4 times in 2 years and so far so good. Within these emails, we made it very clear that I would **not** be able to get the injection done by Wednesday as it was too short notice (*by this time they still hadn't sent the prescription*) and therefore it was looking more and more like we would have to take matters into our own hands and arrange the procedures in the UK.

I spent all Wednesday searching for clinics in the UK who could perform these procedures for me. **Turns out that the ERA test is so specialised, that there are literally only a handful of clinics worldwide that do this test!** *Great!!!* Finally I found the only clinic in the UK who offers the ERA (and the hysteroscopy), Create Health Clinic , but ....drum roll....it was affiliated with IVI in Spain, so probably send the ERA test to them anyway. Not only that, but it was a long waiting list just to get an initial consultation before joining the waiting list for the actual procedures. Just never ending!

In case you are wondering why we are so adamant on doing this ERA (*endometrial receptivity array*)...this test focuses on a woman's optimal timing to receive an embryo and begin the implantation process. Apparently, there is a very small window for implantation and this window is not the same for every woman. Where one woman's optimum receptivity window is on day 16 of her cycle, another woman's could be on day 15 or 18 and this is when embryo transfer should take place. This test is still in the beginning stages of roll-out, explaining why so few clinics have adopted it, but could very well be the reason for repeated implantation failures. As we have had 6 implantation failures, some of those with top quality embryos, then it would be almost madness not to at least try the procedure. We have tried most other, less scientific things, so we just must give this a go!

On Wednesday night, I found what seems like a great clinic in Prague (**with plenty of good reviews!**), Prague Fertility Centre, who also specialise in the ERA test. Yay!. However, they don't do hysteroscopies. *OH come on – why can every IVF clinic not offer every related treatment??!* This meant back to a long waiting list in the UK or use IVI Barcelona.

So (with tail between my legs) I emailed our IVI coordinator asking her weather there is an alternative medicine to take in place of the injection that I could not take on Wednesday so that I could still make the appointment on the 7th. Yes! No problem to take an alternative called Cetrotide apparently, which I could administer myself. *Really?! Why couldn't she tell me this on the same day that I told her we couldn't do the injection at the doctor?* I must take this injection within the next few days depending on my period. Surprisingly she sent me a prescription immediately this time, but now I couldn't get hold of our usual pharmacy in London. I called all Friday morning and sent emails – but nothing. I couldn't believe that the stress had still not ended! I frantically searched the internet again for help (*what would we do without the internet?!?!*). Eventually I found a patient fertility forum that recommended a company called Fertility2U who specialise in rewriting and fulfilling overseas fertility prescriptions. I called them up. They could help but needed a direct email from the clinic within the hour to get it to me the next day. I emailed and called the clinic to make sure that this was done. After an hour and 15 min they sent the whole chain of emails since Sunday to the pharmacy – how unprofessional! But at least (*after paying £230, which included £25 for the prescription rewrite and £25 for next day delivery*), I have the box of injections on my kitchen counter – with no instructions of how to mix the solution and powder. I guess it's a YouTube tutorial for me and a big hope for the best!

So, our flights and accommodation are now booked!! All that remains (*I hope*) is to book a local scan and blood tests for the 31st in preparation for the ERA (fingers crossed!) and learn how to mix injections.

The plan is to get these two procedures done and once the results are in, move on to calmer waters and a clinic that will work **with** me rather than add to the stress that IVF already is!

In the meanwhile, we got back our lab results.

Spermiogram - we are guessing it is normal - just the lab report without any explanation

FISH (sperm genetic test on chromosomes 13, 18 & 21) - Appears to be normal

All standard blood tests - Normal for both of us

Genetic blood tests

Mine have come back as a **C677T MTHFR mutation** with elevated **homocysteine** levels.

Yes, that does look like an abbreviated swear word, and yes, I do say the swear word when I talk about it to Vinny. *How else is one supposed to say it?* I'm barely managing 'hysteroscopy' without a tongue trip.

Well its now way into Sunday evening and time to put all this behind me and move on to a new week filled with love, laughter, fun and opportunity. I will be getting up to some fun this week, which I lock forward to sharing with you all in my next update.

For those of you who made it all the way to the end, well done! Really! Well done!! You are amazing :-).

Love & hugs to you all.

B xxx

Diary Entry 14
This week's Focus: Detox body & mind
Published by Bianca on 26 July 2015

I am happy to report that this week has been a great improvement on the last one. My anxiety levels have gone down and my production has gone up.

This week I have focused on learning more about the *MTHFR gene mutation* and how to change my life now that I know about this mutation. I have researched and researched from one website to 50 others. The amount of information and opinion is overwhelming, as is the extent of the changes people with this gene are expected to make!

The simplest of explanation includes the following summary:

*My body finds it more difficult than other people to eliminate toxins.

*Artificial folic acid (in pill form and within food) and most over-the-counter vitamins are toxic to me.

*Due to this gene mutation, the anti-stress dial in my body is turned right down which means that I am not as equipped as people without this mutation to deal with stressful situations and environments (hence we are prone to strokes and heart attacks!).

*A good dose of **natural** folate (I've been prescribed 5 mgs) and a prescribed multivitamin with high concentrations of **vitamins B2, B6 and B12** is expected to make a world of difference.

Toxins are found in practically everything in the modern (*as well as some things in the natural*) world and it is freaking impossible to avoid them unless one can live completely in nature, living off the land with absolutely no technology or modern amenities.

Ironically, without my computer and mobile phone, which are pumping me with loads of toxins as I use them, I wouldn't know anything about this gene mutation and what products are toxic. The paradox of living in the 21st century!

Not sure why, but my fertility doctor has advised to only start taking this medication after my ERA test and hysteroscopy procedure on the 7th. So, in the meanwhile, I am *slowly* and *with* **as little stress as possible**, starting to implement a few things.

Firstly, I went to the dentist of Friday to inquire about my silver amalgams. I am so sorry for all the sweets and all the other tooth destroying crap I had as a youngster because as a result I have no less than 6 mercury laden fillings! Most of the internet advice has been to have these replaced as they are slowly releasing mercury into my already 'poisoned' system.

However, the dentist informed me that:

-Drilling into my teeth and disrupting the mercury in the fillings **could have a far worse poisoning effect**, as the mercury would then flood my system in a large dose. Even if I replaced one amalgam at a time, each would still emit a higher dose when disturbed as all 6 of them remaining as they are.

-My teeth are currently in good structural condition. Drilling into them to replace one lot of amalgams with another could weaken that structure and contribute to premature tooth loss.

After a few days of thought, I'm leaning toward just leaving them where they are.

How else have I started to detox?

*As my household cleaning products are used up, I am replacing them with more environmentally friendly products which are natural with very little chemicals. I imagine this will be trial and error as I go along.

*I have filled my grocery basket with foods that naturally detox such as, artichokes, asparagus, cauliflower, broccoli, Brussel sprouts, peppers (red, yellow, orange and green), avocados, garlic and berries. Just must remember to wash them well before eating!

*I'm taking advantage of the remaining strawberry season and going to pick my own. My friend, her little dog Monti and I enjoyed a few hours in the fresh air at a local farm filling our containers and bellies with sweet, mouth-watering strawberries. Time spent outside, some socialising, yummy eating and detoxifying the body – not only a productive day but a fun day!

Have a good week everyone!

B xxx

Diary Entry 15
Oh Barcelona
Published by Bianca on 10 August 2015

Today I write to you with longing in my heart. Longing to be back in the wonderful Barcelona with a wonderful husband having a wonderful time and leaving a little of our not so wonderful reality outside of our little world.

We ate. We drank. We shopped (or at least I did). We even visited an ice bar (on the beach) where we put on thermal jackets and gloves for a frosty drink from a glass made completely of ice - and we walked more than 30 000 steps in one day. I know this, because Vinny and I both wear new funky Fitbit watches – the kind that displays our heartbeats, calories burnt, stairs climbed, the distance we have walked and the number of steps we've taken. Together with a Smartphone app and we can also see how many hours of sleep we've had, including the number of times we were restless or awake. This is our new motivation to lose weight and get healthier! So far, it's proving to be a fun gadget and the two of us are constantly glued to our watches like a couple of dorks grilling the other on how many steps they've taken or calories they've eaten. The calorie part doesn't work well when in

Spain!

Our Hilton hotel was perfectly located in the centre of town and getting around was easy on foot and by tram. The weather was fantastically hot, the streets buzzing with summer party people and the night time atmosphere in the Gothic quarter was super charged.

We came very close to missing our flight to Barcelona though. What should have been an hour and a half drive to our airport hotel, took about two and a half hours as we had to stop the car every 15 minutes for me to be sick. Yes, I know…not a pretty picture. We finally got to bed around 2.30 in the morning with the alarm set for 4.45 and then a mad rush to get to the boarding gate by 5.30 – all the way with me chewing on a handful of herbal – herbal!!?? – car sickness tablets combined with a handful of anti-diarrhoea tabs. I was not in a good way at all. The next few hours were horrible with me biting down on my lip and breathing through my teeth, hoping that everything would stay inside at least until we could check into our hotel room. Luckily there was no embarrassing incident.

Thursday my ECG was normal and Friday my hysteroscopy went smoothly. *Sadly, for me it went too smoothly.* I had my hopes on them finding something major to correct which will miraculously 'heal' my infertility. Instead they found everything as good as can be other than the top of my uterine wall which was apparently concave but due to their intervention is now straight. According to the doctor, this does not affect implantation and so means nothing. Truth be told, I feel rather disappointed and defeated with a big chunk of my hope snuffed out.

I do still have a little hope in my ERA test though, the results of which will take 2 to 3 weeks. At that time, we will know whether day 16 of my cycle is my most receptive day for embryo transfer or whether I will need to go through another month of preparation to do the biopsy again.

In the meanwhile, I will try to recover from my surgery as best I can. For some reason the discomfort and bleeding had a delayed reaction. Friday and Saturday, I felt physically great and as much as jumped around the streets of Barcelona! Must have been that air because as soon as we got back home in the early hours of Sunday morning I was struggling, and I have felt horrible ever since.

Wednesday, I have a visit to the breast clinic to check on the 4 excruciatingly painful lumps I have in both breasts. I do feel rather sorry for myself this week and just want a corner to curl up in and someone to hold me, love me, stroke my hair and tell me a funny joke.

On the plus side I have started my MTHFR medication – methylfolate and Vitamin B1, 6 and 12 on the rocks. So, apologies for being Mrs. Morbid this week but hopefully next time I will have bounced back and I'll be doing hoops and somersaults while singing *If you're happy and you know it clap your hands!*

Till then…have a good week everyone

.

Diary Entry 16
IVF is a possessive lover
Published by Bianca on 23 August 2015

Only those of us who have been fighting the war on infertility, and to a small degree those who are close to us, have an accurate understanding of the ugly truth.

Ten years ago, I started the journey of trying to conceive, which escalated into full IVF 2 years ago, resulting in a missed-miscarriage and no less than 6 implantation failures with my own eggs, other people's eggs, my husband's sperm, someone else's sperm – and just nothing! Throughout the entire process, I have been on countless medicines – a variety of hormones, steroids, blood thinners, extra vitamins – you name it. I have had a full range of people with instruments probing, pressing, scratching and observing my (*not so fluffy*) bunny. I have been under anaesthetic 5 times in 2 years and have had as many surgeries. I have been back and forth into forced menopause, then stimulated with daily injections to create hyper youthful ovaries and womb. I have had repeated cycles of dreaming, hoping, wishing, excitement, positive thinking, devastation, disappointment, anger, resentment, jealousy and many moments of wondering just how I was supposed to carry on, how I was supposed to bear being around pregnant women, how I was supposed to endure yet another pregnancy announcement, scan or baby picture on Facebook or walk past the baby aisle biting my lip trying not to break down sobbing, or simply live a life worth living.

During this difficult time in my life, I have a few friends who are there no matter what, but overall, I have become a pariah. Partly my fault, because I have either felt too exhausted, too sick, too sad, too lost, too raw, too broken, too unworthy to be part of the world that is mostly focused on children and family. And partly other 'normal' people's inability to approach me while I have this "disease", from work colleagues to social groups and even friends – but that's a topic for a different day.

My message today is that I am NOT my struggles.
I am NOT my endless conception failures.
I am NOT IVF.

On **Thursday 20 August 2015 at 5pm**, I decided that I am so sick and tired of all things infertility and IVF dominating my life. I am sick and tired of only being associated with infertility – I am a whole, interesting, fun person – I am more than IVF. I am so bored of IVF taking over every conversation – I have more to talk about than just IVF. I am so fed up of IVF controlling every decision I make in my life – I am the master and the captain of this life and – WOW! I DO HAVE A GOOD LIFE!!!

So, I made a list of every negative thing that infertility and IVF have caused in my life, my heart and my relationships, and then I *physically purged* them from my being. I stood up straight and strong in my lounge and one by one

I *pulled* out each agonising ball of searing destruction and pitched each as hard and as far as I could into the universe to deal with…

Inadequacy – Pow! … slip out the back Jack. **My life is more than adequate**.

Exhaustion – hop on the bus Gus!…for far too long I've been stuck in this hamster wheel, running on automatic. **I choose deliberate actions**.

Frustration – no, no, no, make a new plan Stan…finding **acceptance is** finding **peace**

Anger – yes, I admit, I'm angry with infertility – but that's where my anger will *stay, in the back* with infertility and IVF – there's no place for anger **up front in my life** where **love and happiness sit**

Bitterness – run along…**my life is too happy** to entertain you

Jealousy – go join IVF in the back of the bus…I don't need to compare my life to anyone else's, **my life is uniquely and happily mine**

Low self-confidence & low-self-worth – oh please!? Get lost… **I am filled with wonderful gifts to give this world** and whether I have children or not has no bearing on this fact!

Depression – oh you're *evicted*…**This is the house of happiness**

Rawness – go crawling back into the darkness…**it's much too sunny on this street**

Robbed of joy – Ha! Ha!..**laughter is the new black**

Hating my body for failing me – No space for hate here...too much love around. **I love myself.**

Feeling lost – not any more!...I deliberately choose a path that leads to possibility

Tunnel vision – nah uh!...my eyes see only opportunities and wonder

Complaining and whining – **ENOUGH!** ...time to stop being stuck in the same old same old – if you always do the same you will always get the same results

Being a recluse – drop off the key, Lee...**time to get back to the real me!**

I can tell you, it's amazing the weight that lifted from my tired body and worn soul. There is something powerful in using physical actions to boost your mood and gain control over a situation.

Yoga for instance is not only good for your heart, blood flow and stretching the muscles. The fluid movements and deep and slow breathing, bring your mind's focus onto what you are doing, decluttering your thoughts, lowering your stress levels and stimulating a feeling of peace and joy.

You can't deny, that the power in the Haka performed by the All Blacks have had more than a little influence in them being one of the most formidable teams in world rugby!

Then there's the latest craze storming the globe – EFT (emotional freedom techniques) Tapping.

Sound and the movements that create the sound has also been used through the ages in all sorts of therapy – from drumming to chanting, ringing bells, gonging Tibetan singing bowls, clanging symbols and clapping hands.

Why don't you give it a try? Get yourself up, start making some noise, jump around and dispel that negative energy that infertility and IVF has cast over you, so that you can live your life NOW no matter what!

Make your own list, singalong with Paul Simon and get yourself free of that jealous lover.

B xxx

Diary Entry 17
What I Learnt Last Week
Published by Bianca on 11 September 2015

Since my last update, my life has been filled with a mix of days – some busy, some lazy, some filled with the determination to reach my 10,000 steps on my Fitbit, others filled with over-indulging in all the naughty but nice things which then lead me to those hideaway days where I have to pull myself towards myself and get back to a healthy reality. I've had days of extreme frustrations and tears and then those with fun and laughter.

I started writing an update last week Friday and since then it has changed several times as my experiences, reality and my moods have changed. I wanted to write something profound and *'in your face get up and go – banish those demons from your head, kiss the sky and take charge of your life kind of update'.* And then life happened – and I failed to take charge of all the situations (and those that I did take charge of, developed into too much fun to interrupt for writing – although that's not a bad thing hey?). So here I am with no planned masterpiece but simply to tell you what *I* have learnt over the past two weeks:

Life can knock you down and beat you up no matter who you are, where you are, how much you have or don't have, your age, your colour, your race, your career, whether you think you're strong, or brave or positive, or none of those – it just happens and to us all.

When you're down – feel it, cry over it if you need, take some time to feel sorry for yourself, eat the bloody ice-cream with the 4000 calories, have the extra glass of wine, stay in your pyjamas and watch back-to-back films with Charlie Hunnam (or whatever your hunky indulgence is!).

BUT…don't get stuck there. Get up. Dry the tears. Wash the face. Put on those killer heels and red lipstick (figuratively speaking or not – your choice, but a little secret…. it's hard to feel miserable when you're looking good ;-)). Tell those blues to 'Piss off!'. Cut loose the people or situations that have brought you to that level. Seek out the people and situations that make you feel empowered and get back to the YOU that YOU KNOW you really ARE. A mean feminine machine that ROCKS your days and dances to the tunes that YOU have chosen as the theme to your wonderful life. Look back at the crappy feelings to see what you can learn, take the lesson on board and then press 'PLAY'.

And that's it. That's what I learnt last week. That's this week's update.

I hope you are all having a fantastic, purpose-filled, choice-driven life!

B xxx

P.s. Hot and sunny Tampa Bay, Florida awaits me now for 5 weeks of swimming, exploring, eating (sshhhh), fun, love and laughter

Diary Entry 18
Life is Good!
Published by Bianca on 20 October 2015

It's been about 5 weeks since I connected with everyone via my blog updates, but I have a good excuse…I was enjoying the sunshine, the sea, the wildlife and generally the sights, sounds, smells and sensations of Tampa, Florida (with a weekend of Washington DC thrown in for some added spice). The weather was amazing and I spent most of my time outdoors going for long walks along the white sandy beaches of St. Petersburg, swimming, snorkelling with manatees at Crystal River, dolphin watching at every bay, sunset cruising at Clearwater, searching for alligators to shoot with our new purpose-bought zoom lens fully automatic camera, catching up with great friends, eating scrumptious food and tasting rich wines. *With all that to fill my days, can you blame me for taking a leave of absence from the computer?*

What was extra special for me was that while I was having so much fun doing what I was doing, I was reminded of life before endless fertility battles, miscarriage heartbreaks, the disappointments of repeated IVF failures, heaps of pills, injections and a diary filled with clinic appointments and procedures, and I got a taste of what my life could be like whether we have children or not and that taste was very good!

For the first time in years, I didn't have to be Bianca - the poor childless aging infertile woman who bravely tries fighting a disease behind eyes of pain. No, for these few weeks I was Bianca, a fun-loving, adventurous, active, happy woman who was enjoying her holiday to the fullest. I did not need to speak about trying to conceive or IVF or what I should eat or shouldn't drink or whether I should clap my hands three times before standing on my head in the rain while singing a fertility song. None of that mattered. I was having so much fun that the usual cloud of unfulfillment, disappointment and isolation that lurks just behind my exterior gave way to a sparkle that didn't leave room for others to wonder whether there was something missing. Because nothing was (well except for my little furries waiting for me back home).

Yes, I did over-indulge more than I should have and we can't be on holiday all the time, but still, I finally felt what it was going to be like every day if I just broaden my focus and become fully engaged with life and open to all possibilities. I can be Bianca, a fun-loving, adventurous, active woman enjoying all the great things that every day has to offer even while going through fertility treatments, and after failed cycles, whether we never end up getting two lines on a pee stick ever again or whether a couple of transferred embryos decide to stick it through for 30 odd weeks after all – whatever happens, there is always something in life that can and will make me happy if I'm open to it.

That's the problem with women going through fertility treatments – we get so absorbed into the entire process that we spend our lives living outside of life looking in with longing. We get such a bad case of tunnel vision – we will be happy when we have that baby – that we shut ourselves off from the idea of anything else making us happy.

I can't tell you how many times day after day someone writes in one of the fertility support groups,

'That was my last chance at happiness, I don't know how I'm going to carry on with life.'

And

'All I ever wanted was to be a mother, now I'll always just be nothing.'

And

'Life/God/The universe is punishing me for something'.

Or

'Why is life so unfair? I'm a good person.'

And so on and on…I am pretty sure that 99 percent of us on this journey have had similar thoughts at some stage. I most definitely have!

But I have finally grasped the concept of **perception**. Life is all a matter of how you perceive it. If you look for shit, you will get shit. If you look for miracles, you will see them everywhere. If you are going to rely on one thing, such as having that baby to make you happy, then what happens after you have that baby? Then you are not going to be happy until you have another baby – half the women in the support groups who are *'struggling to go on in life'*, are mothers already. Even after another child, your happiness will run out again. *Why?* Because happiness stems from the way you perceive the life you're in. Yes, I agree that life is cruel and unfair and bad things shouldn't happen to good people, but look around you, there are always people who have suffered more than you but are happier than you because they are living and loving life no matter what!

In my IVF news... I have fired IVI Barcelona for lack of professionalism and communication. We are now going with The Prague Fertility Centre, who have found a perfect donor and genetic testing on her has begun to ensure that she is not the carrier of the same 5 genetic diseases that Vinny carries. We are expecting these results in about a month at which time preparations and meds will begin for our next cycle.

Have a great week!

B xxx

Diary Entry 19
What's Your Journey?
Published by Bianca on 11 November 2015

As I have been reading stories about other women on the same road as me, i.e. the fertility journey, something kept popping into my head. Why do they always call this infertility struggle a *journey*? Her journey, their journey, my journey, this journey….almost always the journey is filled with struggling, heartache, frustrations, disappointment…*Isn't a journey supposed to be something good?*

When I look up the word 'journey' in the thesaurus, I find loads of alternative words, most of which are positive:

Adventure – Exploration – Quest – Expedition

Now I don't know about you, but when I think of these words, *I think excitement, fun, joy and energy* – words that I by no means would associate with infertility. Ask my husband – he will tell you that our infertility 'journey' has probably been the least fun he has ever imagined he would ever have in his entire life – and that's the partner who doesn't have to have daily injections, hormonal drugs and repeated surgeries!

So, what then? Do I have an incorrect view of the term 'journey'?

The Oxford Dictionary Online says that a journey is, an act of travelling from one place to another.

Let's see…yes, there sure is a lot of travelling to and from clinic appointments for ultrasound scans to check linings, egg follicles, hormonal levels, egg collections, transfers, betas, etc. But somehow, I don't think that's why we call this thing a journey.

*To try and answer this question, I looked to the second definition of the word 'journey' in the online dictionary…**A long and often difficult process of personal change and development***

Mmmm… that sounds more like it. Is it long? Oh yes! Is it difficult? IS that a trick question? Has it been a process of personal change?

I came to realise not long ago, that this journey is not one from A to Z – from daily injections to daily diapers. Yes, there are several very blessed ladies that do get their 'take-home' baby, but the reality of infertility is that many more will not have the happy ending they have been dreaming of. As I write this, I am moving on to IVF cycle number 8 and its success remains to be seen. If it is not successful, what does this mean for my journey?

Does it mean that many years, and even more tears, empty bank accounts and credit cards, lost friendships or career, more lines on my face and wobbles on my butt, frustrated fights, exhausted days, sleepless nights, heartbreaks, emptiness, missing pieces of myself, depression and runaway self-confidence, and too much more to mention…has all been for nothing? Well that depends on **ME**.

Do I want to be the poor victim of a shitty life, forever living in misery because this big dream I had hasn't come true? Or, do I want to be the empowered hero of my story which is filled with many dreams, endless possibilities and many more ways to bring me happiness?

A brilliant man that once lived, called Nelson Mandela, said,

'There is nothing like returning to a place that remains unchanged to find the ways in which you yourself have altered.'

When you can look at the ways you have changed and could still develop on this journey regardless of whether you take home that baby or not, then you can put the adventure, excitement, joy and fun into your journey.

So, what have I learnt so far?

Wishful thinking is just that – wishful thinking – it gets me nowhere. *What's the alternative?* **Be open to possibilities. Anything is possible! Why limit yourself to specific wishes?**

Thinking positive is over-rated. Thinking positive gets you high for 5 minutes. Positivity is constant mountains and valleys. *What's the alternative?* **Pro-Action!** Get up and **BE** positive. **DO** positive things. Get it out of your mind and into life.

Mantras are for any old puppet. Any ventriloquist's dummy can recite a mantra.

Some people have hundreds of mantras on their wall and still feel depressed every day. It's just lip service. *What's the alternative?* As above – **Pro-Action!** Don't *read* about being the light in someone's darkness. **GO** and **BE** the light.

Gratitude is not an affirmation. Again, I can list hundreds of things every day that I am grateful for, but if I don't FEEL grateful then those lists mean nothing. How do I feel grateful? **BE HAPPY**. If you are grateful for all the loving people in your life, then SHOW them how grateful you are by **BEING HAPPY** around them.

My life is my story. I am unique and so is my journey. *Comparing yourself to others* is the one of the quickest ways to feel ungrateful and unhappy.

Infertility creates self-obsessed, bitter, energy-sapping creatures who no one wants be around. *Is your friend really being a bad friend, or have you just sucked the life out of her? Are you expecting too much from someone who might also be going through her own shit?*

Dreams can be changed at any time! Ok, so maybe I won't be a mother – the dream I've had for the last 20 years but bloody hell, I may have at least another 40 years to go. **I can change the dream! I can have more than one dream. Why limit myself?**

Sometimes you just must **use your common sense**. Do you really think eating 6 brazil nuts instead of 5 or forgetting to stand on your head after sex will spoil your implantation chances? Think realistically. *Why put that kind of ridiculous pressure on yourself?*

I am more than my story. I am a ton of stories. I am not my infertility. Infertility is ONE of many experiences. I am a far more beautiful and complex being. I am not nothing (excuse the double negative) because I don't have children. Being a mother or not being a mother is only one aspect of life.

I **choose** to surround myself only with people and situations that will empower, inspire and encourage me. If anyone else drags me down, it's my own fault.

I control life. Life does not control me. I choose how I WANT to feel and then feel it.

Diary Entry 20
Which Thankfulness Challenge will you take on?
Published by Bianca on 24 November 2015

It's a fact: gratitude = happiness.

We all know the facts but how many of us really embrace the concept of being thankful? ***Gratitude is a feeling – a state of being***, yet I've heard many people rattle off a list of things they say they are grateful for without convincing me or more importantly themselves, that they feel what they are saying. Talk alone doesn't count for all that much. ***The value of being grateful is in our reactions to the feelings that real gratitude instils.***

There are several ways to know if you are really *feeling* grateful:

- Your body will feel *lighter*.
- You will generally feel *healthier* overall.
- Your breathing will be deeper and more *relaxed*.
- Your *posture* will improve as your shoulders will open instead of being hunched, your spine will straighten, and your chin will lift.

- Your lips will default into a *smile*, which will reflect as a sparkle in your eyes.

- You will be more *present* (aware) in what you are doing and with the person or people in front of you.

- You will find a reason to be *happy* with every moment.

- You will *love* the people in your life wholeheartedly, be happy for every new opportunity you have to be with them and be happy simply because they are in your presence.

- Your outlook on life will be from a place of *enough*, rather than a place of lack.

- You will see life's *opportunities and possibilities* in everything around you and in each moment, rather than remaining focused on one obstacle on the road you're travelling.

All of this just from feeling grateful?! Wow! **How amazing that one good state of being can produce so many additional great states of being.**

This week is Thanksgiving week in America, but that doesn't mean that all of us in other parts of the world can't use this week to be thankful too. So come on, let's join and choose which thankfulness challenge we will commit to taking on. Here are some thankfulness challenge ideas…

Brainstorm: write down everything that comes to mind that you feel thankful for. When you are feeling down, negative or angry, take out that piece of paper and read aloud what you wrote until you **really feel** it.

Write a letter to yourself: tell yourself about all the things you are thankful for about yourself. This is something we rarely do but is so important. To love someone wholeheartedly, we need to be able to love ourselves. If we are not compassionate towards ourselves, how can we show compassion to others? If we can't be grateful for things about ourselves, we will struggle to feel grateful for all our other blessings in life.

Start & end your day with thankfulness: every morning before you get out of bed for the day, think, visualise and feel what you could be thankful for going into the day. Do the same at night – think, visualise and feel what you have been thankful for during your day.

A daily gratitude statement: every day on a post-it note, write at least one thing (but there's no limit) that you are thankful for and stick it where you will look at it often – on your computer, fridge, mirror, etc. Really let it sink in and feel it.

Turn a frown upside down: every time you say, write or think something sad, angry or negative – immediately follow it by something you are thankful for and again, don't just say it – feel it.

Thankfulness Christmas Countdown: at the time of writing, it is exactly a month to Christmas, so forget traditional advent countdowns and chocolate-filled little windows, every day from now until Christmas, write down something you are thankful for. Then read them all aloud, either to yourself or share them with your spouse, family and friends on Christmas day.

Which one will you choose?

Happy Thanksgiving week to my American friends.

Diary Entry 21
Empower yourself these holidays with the Power of your Mind
Published by Bianca on 21 December 2015

For the last few months, I have seen several headlines flash across my screen – all with one word in common – *survive*...

"*Survive* thanksgiving" OR "*Survive* Christmas" OR "*Survive* the holidays"

Now, while I have no doubt that these articles mean well and are filled with great tips on coping, I personally refuse to relate to the whole "survivor" mode. To me, the word survivor puts me in victim mode. A survivor escapes a situation whereby she was under someone's or something's control. It's a reaction.

During this fertility journey (and countless other areas and times in my life), I have endured all sorts of heartbreaks and disappointments from which I have had to bounce back and learn to become a survivor.

But I decided that I am MORE than a survivor.

I will no more react to situations – **I will take charge and ACT**.

I am in control and if I am empowered, I won't need to *just* survive.

How do we empower ourselves? **By empowering our minds**.

Napoleon Hill said,

"Whatever your mind can conceive and believe, the mind can achieve regardless of how many times you may have failed in the past."

I can't tell you how many times I read the same sort of posts over and over in the fertility support groups that go along these lines…

'it feels like I'm never going to be a mom…'

'everyone's getting pregnant except me…'

'I just know that I'm going to fail before I even start…'

'I am one of those people who never gets a miracle…'

Does some version of this sound familiar to you? To most of us it will – that's human nature, but we must constantly work at changing our thoughts in order to change our reality.

Everyone knows about **the placebo effect**. This is when a group of people in medicine trials are given the actual medicine, while another group of people are given only sugar pills. Neither group knows which one they have been given. Most of the time the results come back with both groups showing the same reaction. Why? Because their bodies have reacted to whatever they have *thought* they have been given – the real thing or the placebo.

I recently read in a Wayne Dyer book, *Excuses Begone! How to Change Lifelong,*

Self-defeating Thinking Habits, about a surgery experiment. The challenge was to prove that the placebo effect exists in more serious situations like surgery, and not just sugar pills. The patients in the study, all of which had severe knee pain and were referred for knee surgery, were divided into three groups:

Group 1: The surgeon shaved the damaged cartilage in the knee.

Group 2: He flushed out the knee joint and removed material possibly causing the inflammation.

Group 3: This group's surgery was faked. The patients were sedated, and the surgeon made three standard incisions and then talked and acted just like he was performing a real surgery. After 40 minutes, he sewed up the incisions as if he had just completed the surgery.

All three groups were given the same after-care medications and instructions.

The results:

The group with the fake surgeries healed at the same rate and depth as the other two groups. The entire placebo group healed to the point that they were doing all sorts of physical activities that they couldn't do before their "surgery". The placebo patients only found out two years after their "surgery" that it had been a fake. One of the members of the placebo group, Tim Perez, told interviewers, **"In this world anything is possible when you put your mind to it. I know that your mind can work miracles."**

So how about putting a new spin on the holidays? Instead of thinking what you are not, think about what you ARE. *What are you?* I can tell you what I am ...

I AM what I imagine myself to be

I AM living from the perspective of my imagination

I AM living as if my future dream is a present fact in my reality

I AM what I THINK and what I FEEL

I AM open to all possibilities

I AM the best and only the best will come to me

I AM blessed in all areas of my life

I AM healthy

I AM happy

I AM open to all the good in the universe

I AM gentle & kind to myself

I AM worthy of all good things

I AM deserving of miracles

I AM deserving of happiness, joy, confidence and health

I AM trusting the universe to align my imagination, my feelings and my present reality

I AM wonderful and only wonderful things happen to me

Now, I am one of the most sceptical people when it comes to mantras. And that's because it's easy to rattle off a bunch of words without letting them truly register in your heart and mind. No matter how dedicated you are to repeating your mantras every day, even twenty times a day, *if you don't feel the words then you are just making a noise and wasting your time.*

Think of someone you really love. Think of the way you feel when you tell them that you love them. How powerful is that feeling?! **That's the kind of feeling that you need to feel from your mantras. FEELING is the key** here. **What you think AND FEEL will become your reality.**

Meditate on that over the next week, start putting it into practice and I'm positive that you won't need to scrape through the next few weeks as merely a survivor!

HAPPY HOLIDAYS!

B xxx

Diary Entry 22
It's National Fertility Week & Our 8th IVF Fail
Published by Bianca on 26 April 2016

Two weeks ago our IVF journey came to an end after our 8th IVF failed.

30th of January, I had surgery on my tubes and ovaries – a laparoscopy to remove stage 2 endometriosis and a cyst. From what we have been told and through my own research, we understand that any amount of endometriosis – from stage 1 to 4, could negatively affect fertility. It was a rough operation for me. I kept drifting in and out of consciousness after the surgery. My body freaked out – I kept throwing up, I overheated and my blood pressure plummeted. I was on liquid paracetamol and diluted morphine for a few days, and strong codeine for the next two weeks. I could barely walk, and the pain was excruciating for at least two weeks. However, at the time it was all worth it as it gave me a glimmer of hope that eliminating the endometriosis and the cyst would make way for an embryo to finally attach and grow into a healthy baby inside my womb.

Sadly this was not the case. This was not our magic button. In fact, we warned that they endo will keep growing back because that is the nature of endometriosis. It comes back again more aggressively and judging by the monthly pain, I have no doubt it's already growing back. At £5000 an operation to remove it, it looks like it is here to stay. So, that's that. It's over.

This has been a 3 year journey (*not counting the many years of trying and testing and probing and heartache <u>before</u> the actual IVF even began*)…of excitement, elation, devastation, hope, fear, raging hormones, nausea, anxiety, tears, darkness, isolation, breath-holding, probing, injections, pill-popping, dangerously low blood pressure, over-heating, throwing up, liquid paracetamol, codeine, morphine, stress, love, commitment, strength, discovery, frustration, worry, grief, amazement, gratitude, exhaustion, pain, IV drips, catheters, empty bank balances, maxed credit cards, desperate loans, dreams, determination, apprehension, operations, craziness, kindness, friendship, madness, herbs, acupuncture, vitamins, teas, optimism, pessimism, fights, rejection, tenderness, uncertainty, screams, yearning, admiration, bitterness, jealousy, defeat, compassion, despair, sorrow, doubt, honesty, inspiration, change, growth, love and everything else in between.

I've lost friends along the way. Those that avoided me because *my* fertility struggles made *them* uncomfortable. Others were blatantly cold and insensitive, not understanding how the constant hormones controlled all my moods or made me physically sick and mentally and emotionally drained or how my consuming misery left me feeling completely worthless in a world where motherhood is constantly celebrated – where child creation and birth is considered the ultimate gift that a woman can offer to the universe – where a woman's stretchmarks and scars are a mark of her beauty simply because they mean that she carried and gave life. *What about my stretchmarks and scars – the ones I developed from 3 years of non-stop fertility drugs, treatments and operations? What about the scars on my heart and my soul? The ones that will forever remind me of what I sacrificed for something that never happened?*

But that's ok…because I have learnt the true value of friendship, love, kindness, sacrifice, compassion and living.

On my one side I have a handful of dedicated angels of family and friends, who have been holding my hand and my heart in spirit even when not in the physical (*I hope you know who you are. I have appreciated every word, every gesture, every smile, every hug, every heart emoji. Thank you so much. I love you guys*).

And on the other side I have made amazing new friendships with the most incredible, brave, gorgeous, wonderful and inspirational women, who have changed my life for the better just by being in it. These women have made me appreciate all the good things I already have in my life. These women have given me the strength to go out and be what and who I want to be in my life despite the challenges I face. These women shine a light for others when they need it most and they have never failed to be there in my darkest times. These women have become warriors not victims of their circumstance.

These are women who should all be celebrated during this week – National Fertility Awareness Week in the USA – and every week, whether they have attained their dreams of motherhood or not. To all of you sensational women in my support groups, I thank you, I love you and I appreciate you – thank you for being with me on this journey and for making me a better version of me every day.

I will be ok.

Vinny, my magnificent, one-in-a-million soulmate, whom I love with all my being, and I, will be ok. No, we will be **more** than ok. We will be exceptionally good.

. This might be the end of the IVF road, but this is not the end of of the journey called life, filled with endless possibilities of all things good. Maybe this is the end of motherhood but it is not the end of *womanhood*. I am 100% woman and I will celebrate that every day!

This week might be filled with tears for me, for our loss, for my fellow women in the same scenario and their loss but next week I will take a deep breath, put on my red heels and dance for joy and gratitude, because my life is awesome and I am a fucking awesome woman!

And moving to Florida helps a tad too ha ;-). On that side note, yesterday I was blessed to see a manatee come up for air right in front of me as I sat in our gardens overlooking the bay. I firmly believe that if we ask the right questions, nature provides the answers. Manatees are slow, trusting, gentle, peaceful creatures and my message is to move slowly through my emotions, feel them, then leave them behind and move on as I trust in my path, my senses and the universe to provide new opportunities for me.

And just for something a little extra… this is one of my all-time favourite ballads that has always filled me with peace and dreams of endless possibilities.

Love B xxx

In the silence of the darkness, when all are fast asleep.

I live inside a dream calling to your spirit.

As a sail calls the wind, hear the angels sing.

Far beyond the sun, across the western sky,

Reach into the blackness find a silver line.

In a voice I whisper, a candle in the night.

We'll carry all our dreams on a single beam of light.

Close your eyes, look into the dream,

Winds of change will winds of fortune bring.

Fly away to a rainbow in the sky. Gold is at the end for each of us to find

There the road begins where another one will end

Here the four winds know who will break and who will bend.

All to be the master of the wind.

Falling stars now light my way.

My life was written on the wind.

Clouds above, clouds below,

High ascend the dreams within.

When the wind fills the sky, the clouds will move aside

And there will be the road to all our dreams.

For any day that stings two better days it brings.

Nothing is as bad as it seems.

Close your eyes, look into the dream.

Winds of change will winds of fortune bring.

Fly away to a rainbow in the sky, gold is at the end for each of us to find.

There the road begins where another one will end.

Here the four winds know who will break and who will bend.

All to be the master of the wind.

Manowar – Master of the Wind

Diary Entry 23
There WILL be a Bun in the Oven...Just Not This Oven
Published by Bianca on 27 July 2016

It's been a while since my last heart to-heart with you guys.

Since then I have been living it up in our new home of Florida. I have been getting my Vitamin SEA, talking to the local wildlife – dolphins, manatees, herons, crows, sharks, my neighbours' awesome dogs – all in my back yard, partying with new good friends, getting a tan, swimming...I started a new job, I published a book and I've looked into other options to create our much wanted family.

3 Months ago, when our 8th IVF failed, my hubby and I agreed to stop the treatments. It has been too many years of hormones, steroids, injections, operations, probing, pricking, nausea, hope and despair was finally enough for us.

However, that innate feeling of wanting to have a family wouldn't budge and we couldn't simply ignore it. So began my exploration into **Surrogacy**. I grieved for the loss of my own eggs in December 2014. I grieved for that elusive feeling of having a child grow and develop within my own body in April this year. But fuck it, at this stage I am refusing to grieve for empty arms or for the loss of joy that children would bring to our lives. **We will be parents one way or another and right now that way is looking good for Surrogacy!**

After extensive research, we have decided to go with an agency in Ukraine. In a nutshell it comes down to favourable surrogacy laws that protect the intended parents, cost and unlimited number of tries until we bring home our baby. **Yes!!!** No matter how many times we transfer embryos to one or more surrogates, we won't stop until we have our baby in our arms – at NO extra cost!

There is one catch…Vinny's sperm has got to be top quality for us to qualify for this guarantee offer. This means that with immediate effect, my dear husband has stopped all alcohol, dairy, wheat, gluten, sugar, soy, processed foods and trans fats. Instead he must fill his body with good sperm-building nutrients and supplements. He has also cut out as many sperm killers as possible such as plastic, chemicals, heat and tap water. These lists are long and tough and he needs to follow them for close to three months, which is how long it takes sperm to regenerate and mature.

It's rather strange being the one on the other side. My husband is finally having a walk in my shoes (*well, kind of – minus all the hormones, steroids and operations*) while all I need to do is jump up and down with excitement, counting down the days until our initial consultation to get the ball rolling in Kiev, Ukraine middle of October!!!!

I love him even more for this. He is the best future daddy that this future mamma could want!

Let's wish him luck!!! Here's to a Mini Vinny :)!

Speak soon everyone.

Love to you all.

B xxx

Diary Entry 24
The Countdown has begun...Please help cheer for my hubby's swimmers!!!
Published by Bianca on 10 October 2016

The day of reckoning is finally drawing closer!!!

It's been 3 months of (mostly...it's been a little difficult towards the end) being good following a diet and lifestyle of ...

ONLY ORGANIC food products, vitamin B6, B12, Selenium, CoQ10, vitamin E, L'Carnitine, Alpha Lipoic Acid, American Ginseng, Zinc, Ashwaganda and Maca Root, melatonin, beef, turkey, lamb, peanut butter, spinach kale, sweet potatoes, cranberries, sunflower seeds, nuts, coconut oil, filtered water, as little chemicals as possible (*this includes all toiletries and household products and cookware – we use only glass, silicone and cast iron*).

Regular exercise and good sleep.

AND

NO alcohol, wheat, dairy, sugar, processed foods, fats (*other than coconut and* *olive oil*), coffee, plastics, register receipts, – and, he says, no fun ha ha.

There's probably loads more that he's doing that I'm forgetting right now. In any case, it was a major shift for someone who loves processed & junk food, hates taking tablets and before this, couldn't have given two hoots about the chemicals we are exposed to. **I am VERY VERY PROUD of my hubby and he floored me by showing so much commitment and determination in following through on his part in (hopefully) getting us our baby. I can't thank him enough for doing this for us!**

On Saturday 15 October, we fly from Tampa to Ukraine to have our first consultation with our chosen clinic for donor egg & surrogacy. The hubby will give several deposits and if they are top quality, we will be confirmed for our 'baby-guarantee' package. This means that we will get a take-home baby even if it means going through several egg donors and surrogates (at no extra charge) until we have success. Everything at this stage is riding on those swimmers.

So, please take out your pom poms and start cheering for us!!! After many years, 8 failed IVF cycles, multiple heartbreaks and oceans of tears, we are urging the universe to finally provide us with the family that we long for. Please send us as much positive energy as you can magic together!

B xxx

Diary Entry 25
A Silver Medal for My Hubby's Swimmers – Surrogacy here we come...
Published by Bianca on 18 October 2016

Hi Everyone!

As you can probably tell from the title, our first consultation at our new clinic in Ukraine was a success! Whooooo hooooo!!!! The embryologist said that she can "totally work with" Vinny's sperm. **We have signed our unlimited try/baby guarantee contracts and the search for our egg donor and surrogate has begun!!**

Vinny's strict diet has worked! YAY!!!!

We have been given access to an online portal with 240 egg donors to choose from (many of whom look very similar to me!) and **we have been advised that we could find a surrogate within a month – then it's all systems go!!**

We have met super people – a wonderful couple from Australia who we clicked with straight away and who will be our cycle/surrogate buddies throughout this new and exciting journey. This journey brings together like-minded people who become life-long friends!

All-in-all, a fantastic experience so far and more great things to come. Here's to a 2017 Smith baby (or twins!)!

Diary Entry 26
Countdown to (donor) Egg Collection with our
Surrogate ready & waiting...
Published by Bianca on 21 October 2016

Hi Friends!

This is just a quick one to share the exciting news that we received today...We have a donor and we have a surrogate...both are syncing their cycles as we speak and egg collection is set for 9 November – less than 3 weeks away !!!!!!!!! I can't even describe how excited we are!!!!!! If all goes according to plan, our surrogate could have a confirmed pregnancy by end November and we could be parents by end July/August 2017 !!!!!!!!!!!! Fingers and toes and everything crossed. Please keep cheering us on, lovely people.
More updates about our experience here in Ukraine will follow soon.

Love to you all, B

Diary Entry 27
Ukraine Adventures
Published by Bianca on 31 October 2016

Hi Again Friends!

Well, we are back in Tampa from our first visit to Ukraine. It was a great week despite the cold and being over-fed by our housekeeper...some serious exercise and healthy eating required ASAP!

Yes, part of our package included an apartment with a driver and a live-in housekeeper, who cleaned, did our washing, shopped and cooked three huge meals a day as well as supplied a bottomless bowl of chocolates and sweets!

All of these were not needed in this first visit but will prove very helpful when we are back there for baby's birth and need to remain in Kiev for 3 months while the paperwork is sorted. Yip, 3 months is how long it takes the UK government to process the paperwork for internationally born surrogate babies.

But there's still some time until that happens (at least 9 months ;-)), so back to the present…here's a little summary of our trip…

Ukraine Experience

* **Cold!!!** It sounds like an exaggeration, but it really felt like the temp dropped a bit more every day that we were there. The first two days we had blue skies and sunshine and I thought, wow, what beautiful weather – not cold at all. Then, I lost the feeling in my hands and face and my body slowed down to a deathly pace (ok maybe a little exaggeration, but still too cold for my lips to even say brrrrrrrr!)

* **Vodka!!!** The supermarkets had aisles and more aisles of vodka in every shape of bottle, with a cost that started as little as $1.50 for a litre.

* **Architecture** – there are many beautiful buildings in Kiev, specifically churches and golden domes.

* **Food** includes hearty meals to keep you warm – vegetable and meat soups, bread, potatoes (with EVERY meal), pasta, cheese dishes, dumplings, pizza style omelettes and pies. It's extremely filling and heavy for us that are used to things like salads and minimum starch. There are several coffee shops, restaurants and mobile food stalls all along the roads.

* **Language** – Ukraine does not use the Roman alphabet and that makes it difficult to decipher and guess at. It has 33 letters, most of which look more like drawings or symbols to us and unless you have studied the language, you would have no idea how to pronounce it. Getting lost in town (as we did a few times) can be a little scary when you cannot read the names of the street or ask anyone for directions. Not many people speak English. Communicating with our housekeeper was with Google Translate and even then, there were definite sentiments and phrases lost in those translations.

Unfortunately, this made it more than challenging to get to know our housekeeper beyond telling her what time we wanted our next meal.

* **Things to see & do** – because we were only there for a short time while knowing that we would be back again, and because I was not doing too well in the cold, we didn't go out and about much.

We walked around the town centre for a bit exploring the tourist square which is filled with a variety of 'acts' to attract money – acrobatics, street dance, animal attractions, men in animal suits – we got pounced upon by a clever but funny bloke in a bear suit who made a good $30 from us in 10 minutes for taking pictures with him – which we didn't want in the first place! He did give us a laugh at least.

A good way to get our general bearings of the city, was the Kiev city tour bus. It travels past 11 city attractions where you can also get off and explore if you choose to. The full tour is about 2 hours long and costs less than 10 US Dollars a ticket. ** A little tip here…try not to drink too much before getting on the bus tour as the nearest toilet might be in one of the parks where you will find a hole in the ground in place of a toilet – and yes, that's both on the men's and women's sides – but I was desperate after 2 large Irish coffees that I had to have for warmth!

A great restaurant and bar (recommended by one of my friends) is the Buddha Bar. Beautiful decor, atmosphere, food (we had quality sushi), lounge and DJ.

Karaoke bars are everywhere, but we didn't try one of them even though my hubby loves to grab the mic at a karaoke. We thought perhaps it might be difficult singing in Ukrainian!

We also heard that the Thai massage is excellent and only costs around 40 US Dollars for 2 hours!

* The **cost of things** is way cheaper than the UK and USA. This goes for food, drinks, taxis and clothes, including designer items.

Fingers crossed for a great number of quality eggs and embryos on 9 November!!!

Happy Halloween! Have a great day/ evening! Xxx

Diary Entry 28
Now begins the 2ww – the longest wait in history – will we be preggers or not?!
Published by Bianca on 14 November 2016

Hi Everyone!

I promised an update soon after our egg donor's egg collection on the 9th of November and I finally have some news to report…so here's just a quick message to say…….

Our clinic confirmed that embryo transfer to our surrogate today was a success!
They collected 9 eggs, 6 fertilized and 3 made it to day 5 transfer. I believe they were AA grade – which is really good!

Pregnancy test is in 2 weeks. They won't give me the exact date, only that they will contact me in 2 weeks with the result. *Sigh* I'm going to be on the edge of my seat until then!!!!

Friends, please send me all the positive vibes and good magic you can muster for a positive result. This month marks 3 years since we went for our devastating 12-week scan at which we discovered that our little one's heart had stopped. How fitting would it be to get a positive result at this very time?!

Update again in 2 weeks! I will be spending that time trying to find my calm centre and just breathe!!

B xxxx

Diary Entry 29
Why is 2367 a Magical Number for us?
Published by Bianca on 29 November 2016

Hello Friends!

Due to the fact that my in-laws and my dad are visiting from the UK and Germany for 2 weeks and we are doing the touristy thing, this will be short, but I just had to share…

2367 is the level of pregnancy hormone that is present in our surrogate's blood stream – nice and HIGH! Yes…we are PREGNANT!!!!!!!!!!!!!!!!!!!!!!!! Her first scan is in 2 weeks at which time they will confirm a definite uterine pregnancy and how many embryos took – we transferred three and are hoping for twins – fingers and toes crossed!!!!

On this day 3 years ago, we found out at our 12-week scan that our little baby's heartbeat had stopped. It was the most devastating moment of our lives. How awesome to receive the wonderful news that we are have another shot at being parents. Words cannot describe how elated we are! WOW!!!!!!!!!

Thank you so much to all of you for always cheering us on – we are so blessed to have all your good energy in our lives.

All our love,
B&V xxxx

Next update after our surrogate's scan…

p.s I got a new tattoo a few days ago of a cat riding a unicorn with a rainbow in the background…because I never want to stop believing in magic!

Diary Entry 30
Donor + Surrogate + Dad + Wannabee Mom = 2 Mini Vinnies !!
Published by Bianca on 14 December 2016

Hey Friends…

Well it's been quite an exciting day in my world :).

I lay awake all night waiting for the all-important report on our surrogate's viability ultrasound – is it a proper uterine pregnancy? Is there a heartbeat? Is it measuring what it should? And of course…how many embryos implanted after transferring 3 grade AA's ?!?!
I'm sure you've guessed by now by the title of this post, that 2 heartbeats were confirmed, each with their own little sac measuring what they should at 6 weeks. Phwew!!!! Sigh of relief and of course all-day jumps of excitement!!!!!

Yes, it's still early and we have a lot of milestones to pass yet, but this is the first December in 3 years that I feel happy enough to celebrate the holidays :).

This was my Facebook post from 3 years ago to the day – how bizarre is that!!! – after we had the most devastating 12-week ultrasound and discovered our baby's heart had stopped…

"I don't know how I'm going to get through the 'festive season'. The last thing I have the emotional strength for is to be festive. Just want to go to sleep today and wake up in February (to begin our next IVF cycle). Can't even manage a few days without crying."

Today I have tears of joy and renewed hope, thanks to the incredible opportunity of using a surrogate.

It's taken a while, but finally I feel happy enough to welcome the festivities with confidence that our family dreams are materialising in this world here and now :). That mamma feeling is digging in and digging firm :). And as I keep telling my friends, every cloud has its glittery lining…we are 6 weeks pregnant with twins and I'm getting toasty on bubbly ha ha. I might have a hangover that will last a few hours but no morning sickness, no moods, no silly cravings, no pushing and no stretchmarks…
So, who's got the better end of the stick?!

Happy Holidays beautiful people and thank you always for your amazing support and invaluable friendship … speak soon, Love B xxx

Diary Entry 31
We've Made it to 13 Weeks With Our Two Mini-Vinnies!
Published by Bianca on 31 January 2017

Hey Friends.......!

This is not going to be a long post because I'm just too excited to form coherent words, but I must document this huge milestone! This is the absolute farthest that we have come to having our much loved and wanted family! All thanks to the amazing gift of surrogacy!

The report just came in this morning that our twin **BOYS** are looking good! They are measuring 13 weeks and due 7 August. Although this is a due date for a singleton, and they say that twins are very often a 3 to 4 weeks earlier so who knows what will happen...we just have to be ready!

So, it's twin shopping time....first on the agenda, a twin mommy car. Also, I need to brush up on my Russian (*by brush up, I mean learn it from scratch*) for my 3 months I'm going to be spending in Ukraine when they are born. Any volunteers?

Well I'm all over the place right now – walking on clouds in a daze, so I might just end it there for today.

Thank you to everyone that has always been a wonderful support to us over the years of heartbreak. I wouldn't have had the strength to make it this far without you all.

Of course, I won't be calm until our little bundles are healthy and safe in our arms but it's a great start isn't it?!

Next scan is due in about a month.

Love to you all.

B xxx

Diary Entry 32
Our Boys Are Growing – 18 Weeks today
Published by Bianca on 1 March 2017

Hi Friends!

Many people on my Facebook friends list will already have got my update and scan pics of our boys yesterday as I was too excited to keep them to myself until I had some time to blog.

Bottom line ... they are looking too gorgeous and growing well with no health concerns so far :).

I am sooo in love with them already and can't wait to kiss their little faces and give them loads of cuddles! Baby boy 1 seems to be all legs like his daddy (who is 6 foot 4) ha ha.

Vinny and I decided to go out for dinner last night to celebrate this amazing milestone (*it's so important to always celebrate every great moment*) and we discovered that it is mardi gras week in the USA. One of our favourite restaurants in our area had a mardi gras special meal which included a tasty cake for dessert – King Cake it's called.

We had a little giggle in the beginning because our host told us that the tradition was to put a little baby in the middle of the big cake and whichever patron of the restaurant gets the slice with the baby in it, gets a free drink – we giggled because obviously we were celebrating our babies progress on the same day that they were doing this 'baby' cake. Imagine how hard we laughed when we actually got the baby in our slice of cake that Vinny and I shared!!!

What are the odds in a full restaurant on the day we were celebrating our babies?!? Is that a sure confirmation or what!?

Thank you for sharing in our joy guys!

Till next time…
Lots of love,
B xxx

Diary Entry 33
Letter One to My Twin Boys
Published by Bianca on 29 March 2017

My gorgeous boys,

This is my first letter to you two. It's not quite the beginning of our story, but there isn't really a beginning – because since the beginning of this time and the time before that and even way, way back, we (your mom and dad) have had you both in our hearts and spirit. You two are our spirit babies and soon you will be our babies in the physical world too. We don't know why you were not able to get to us in the traditional way, but that does not matter at all – we are just as excited to connect with you and in just a few months, to kiss your cute, little new born faces. We love you so much already.

Tomorrow, our surrogate, your human incubator in Ukraine, will officially be 22 weeks pregnant with you both. Thursday she is due for an updated ultrasound to make sure that you are both growing and developing just as you should.

This moment in time – a few days before our update from the clinic – is both exciting and terrifying. After everything we have been through to get you to this point, we are still walking on a dream and we are breathing ever so gently to ensure that the dream doesn't blow away in the mist.

We have done our very best to shine the brightest light for you two to follow home to us. And we will continue to do our best for you both each moment of each day as long as we live. On my shoulders I have sabotaging little leprechauns muttering in my head, giving me all sorts of fears and anxieties, trying their best to make me doubt my worthiness to receive these blessings but I know in my heart and in my spirit that our love for you will bring you both safely to our arms at the right time in just a few months.

So, armed with this knowledge, I refuse to give in to the saboteurs but instead, I will do my happy dance in anticipation of seeing your gorgeous little 3D pictures and hear your strong little heartbeats. We can't wait to meet you two amazing little boys in person very soon!

Love your mom (and dad) <3 xxx

Diary Entry 34
Letter Two to My Twin Boys
Published by Bianca on 6 April 2017

My gorgeous boys,

It's been a week since we've had another glimpse of your sweet little faces on the 22-week ultrasound.

We have been assured that you are both well and growing as you should. Daddy has a feeling that you are going to be big boys like him. This past weekend we went to browse around a warehouse of baby stuff – the bug has bit and now that we have started buying things for you, it's difficult to stop – and your dad said we should just skip the new born sizes as he's convinced that you're going to be born already needing size 6 months – ha ha, he's so funny, you'll discover that soon enough.

Your daddy is sooo excited to have you here. He can't stop talking about all the things you three are going to do together – camping, fishing, roller coasters (all the stuff mommy doesn't like to do). Right from the start, he always said that we were having boys and my eyes nearly popped into the back of my head when I read the first reports confirming that you two were in fact boys. He smiled smugly, all-knowing. Daddy's superheroes! He has already picked out little Batman-style baby walkers and if he has his way, every outfit you two wear from birth until you decide for yourself what to wear, will be one or other superhero.

Four months until your due date (unless you decide to escape earlier than you should) and I can't stop thinking about you. I am trying to get a business into place before you arrive but it's so hard to concentrate when all I want to do is *baby stuff*. After so many years to get right here right now, I just want to bathe in this happiness every minute of every day.

Love your mom (and dad) <3 xxx

Diary Entry 35
Letter Three to My Twin Boys
Published by Bianca on 17 April 2017

Hey My Two Boys,

It's your mom again. It's been nearly 3 weeks since our last ultrasound update and I'm counting down until the next one. We don't have a date yet but I'm guessing it will be toward the end of the month.

Today is an emotional one for me and the tears are flowing like whisky at a wake. For the first time in this surrogacy journey, I've been hit with the sadness stick.

Sadness for not being able to carry you in my own body.

Sadness for not being able to show off my growing belly and be told how lovely I look with that pregnant glow.

Sadness for not being able to feel you moving around and giving me little kicks.

Sadness for not being able to swap pregnancy stories with my pregnant friends.

Sadness for not being able to walk next to a proud daddy during the day who puts his head on my belly and talks to you at night.

Sadness for not having everyone look at me and congratulate me for our coming happiness – instead when I tell them that we are expecting twins they look at my flat belly like I'm crazy – or when I walk around the baby shops, the staff automatically assume that I am buying baby gifts for friends instead of us.

Sadness that this is the week that babies start identifying their mom's voices and I'm not there for you to hear mine. I'm not there to put earphones onto my belly and play music or read to you or connect in any way until you are born.

Sadness that in order to breast feed, I will need to take a bunch of hormones to cheat my body into thinking that I am pregnant so that it can produce milk – how emotionally cruel – to be pregnant without actually being pregnant (and then still most induced lactation doesn't produce enough milk anyway).

Sadness for us having to go to extremes to bring you here with us. But still, I am so grateful for the miracle of surrogacy so that we can get you here at all!

Sadness that by UK law I am not considered your mother until I adopt you through the high court who must decide whether I am worthy of loving you and caring for you.

I am not writing this to make you or anyone else feel sad. I am writing to reset myself and connect with you in the only way I can right now – and I already feel better for my spirit connecting with the two of yours and sending you both love that transcends everything on this earthly dimension.

112 days until your due date...when the sunshine in my heart will match the sunshine outside.

Don't you worry, by the time of my next letter, I will have picked myself up like I always do. If there's one thing you can learn from your mom and dad, it's to keep rising above.

Love your mom (and dad) <3 xxx

Diary Entry 36
Letter Four to My Twin Boys
Published by Bianca on 31 May 2017

To My Darling Boys,

Today is one of excitement as we draw closer to your arrival!

This morning we met your carrier for the first time over skype. Your dad and I woke up at 3am so that we could be alert enough to speak to her at 4am (through an English/Ukrainian translator). Here in Florida, we are 7 hours behind in time so a little tricky to coordinate, but you could say that we are already preparing for the sleepless nights we keep hearing that we will have when you get here ;-).

How do you two big, growing boys manage to make our surrogate look so small and cute?! We expected to see you two spreading out all over the place, leaving no room for your poor carrier to move or breathe even. Instead you two are tucked comfortably into a neat little ball. We did learn that you two are little busy bees who can't keep still. It's a good thing that your dad and I are relatively active ourselves, as I have a feeling we will be doing many miles of chasing you all over the apartment, the garden, the beach, the shops…and chasing after you chasing after the kitties. Those furry little girls have no idea what's coming into their lives … aren't they in for a treat!? We hope that you love them and all animals as much as we do – we will certainly help you to see the beauty in all the earth's creatures.

It feels like forever between ultrasound updates. Today you are measuring 30 weeks and 2 days and already weighing 4 pounds (1.8 kgs) – a nice fat jump since the last time :). And you look cuter and cuter. We just can't wait until you are in our arms!

I have washed all your little clothes that we have bought to take with to Kiev, attended a great course on the first year with twins, we are busy reading and double reading a stack of new parent books, have an infant CPR class booked before we leave and your dad has promised that this weekend he will continue the transformation of his office into your room – finally! He has no idea how exciting it is for a future mama to create the perfect space for her babies. I have spent days trying to find just the right things to make your room feel comfy, safe and joyfully dreamy, but where, most importantly you will always feel an energy of total love.

Oh, and I must tell you…every year when Mother's Day comes around, my heart is broken over and over and I spend this day sobbing, wishing and dreaming of what always escapes me – being a mother. Well, of course this year is different! You two are living in our surrogate's womb and soon you will be with us. No more depressing Mother's Days. From now on we plan to celebrate this special day with you our beautiful boys. So, guess what your (not usually very romantic or creative) dad did? He gave me a beautiful Mother's Day card from the womb! He printed out pictures of your gorgeous little faces from our last ultrasound and created a lovely card from it. I was so surprised that I nearly swallowed the card!

See you again at your next ultrasound end of June – counting the days already!!!

Love your mom (and dad) xxx

Diary Entry 37
Day 2 in Kiev, Ukraine – Prepping for our Surrogate Twin Boys
Published by Bianca on 9 July 2017

I know that its been a while since I've updated you guys on our baby preparations, but it's been crazy busy trying to get everything ticked on our to-do-lists before being away for 4-5 months with new born babies in a foreign country. Extreme excitement, arranging to get my furry girls well-taken care of while we're away, getting a business in place which I can (maybe) do remotely while the babies are napping, organising all the paperwork, packing -unpacking-repacking, shopping for the boys, and preparing mentally and emotionally for their arrival has left no time for blogging.

In the meanwhile, I started a video channel on You Tube. The aim is to vlog about our adventures as new surrogate twin parents. I'm not sure at this stage where it will all lead – it might go nowhere, it might be complete baby spam, or it might be something interesting to the masses – who knows at this stage?

I'm not a natural in front of the camera and these videos are totally amateur, but feel free to have a look. Here's the link to my channel **youtube.com/channel/UCZikz9DFQIYQ5uR3Am8Kq6A** where you can find everything from chatting to you about our preparations for the boys – their nursery, where we live, the first leg of our trip to meet our boys – UK and a side interview I did with a US surrogate about her journey. ** *(extra note… at time of publishing this book, my channel is filled with 2 years of baby/toddler spam!)*

back to the present:

Today started with a healthy breakfast of fruit and yogurt. It could easily be 3 cooked meals a day prepared by our housekeeper, but that would be dangerous! So instead we went for the light fare and then mapped out our route to find all the baby shops in the area. Soon, armed with the phone's GPS for comfort, we set off full of adventurous spirits.
It was a beautiful, sunny day with just the right temperature for shorts and a summery T. Not far from our apartment, we walked through a gorgeously green park with pathways, children's play area and a little skyway obstacle course of zip lines and rope bridges.

There are many parks connected via pedestrian tunnels and this is where we saw something that neither of us had seen before – a young (slight) lady pushed a baby stroller down these sleeper type contraptions with the wheels balancing on either side. Once through the tunnel, she reversed herself and her stroller up the sleepers again! Then we started noticing these everywhere around the city. Quite an ingenious idea, but I'm not so sure if I could prevent myself tumbling and crumbling into a heap at the bottom, babies and all! Hubby says I'm just going to have to practice – good to know he has so much faith in my balancing abilities!

We visited a baby shop, called Antoshka, where we were followed around by the staff like we were suspected criminals. It might have been the tattoos. A woman with tattoos in Ukraine was not something seen every day and of course I have more than a few.

An hour and a half walk from our apartment, we finally arrived in the city centre. Here we had lunch was in the town square at the Karaoke Bar – a feast for a King. That's when Vinny decided that a run every night in the park at our apartments was needed if he was going to still fit into his clothes by the time we go home.

The town square is tourist central, and like any tourist area, it is filled with all sorts of entertainers trying to get visitors to dig deep into their pockets. Last year we were scammed by the Ukrainian Bear (*a very clever salesman in a giant bear suit who managed to politely take every bit of cash from our pockets*). This time we decided not to be conned again...until...the Pigeon Men told their 4 pet pigeons to hop on our shoulders for photos. It took a lot of energy to finally get away with promises of returning to bring them Dollars or Pounds. We gave them all the Ukrainian money we had but their hearts were set on our currencies. Vinny is going to try his best to avoid the square from now on. I feel bad and might sneak back with some currency some time next week. The pigeon's expression in the one photo had me in stitches and is so worth going back to give them Pounds just for that :)!

My clever hubby navigated the Metro for us with ease and we have decided that will probably be our main mode of transport when out and about. A one way ticket (or green token that looks like something out of a box of compendium games) to anywhere around the city, is 4 Hryvnia – you put in a 20 Hryvnia note and you get 5 tokens (77 cents US / 60 pence UK for 5 trips!!). We discovered that it is crazy busy during the week and very suffocating! *Not a good idea with newborns, as you just don't know what you can pick up in there!! Best to stay away and either walk or catch an Über. Also, something we learnt the other day, is that you can still pay cash for an Über and it is much cheaper than a taxi!*

On our walk back to the apartment we came across a colony of feral cats. Now, I am one major Cat Lady, so for me this is a bittersweet encounter. Sweet, because oh my goodness, they are just too beautiful and there are a group of juveniles, probably around 6 months old that I just want to cuddle and bring home. Bitter, because they are outside which is all very well in the summer but it pains me to think how they survive the bitterness of the long and extreme Ukrainian winter (temps often plummet to -30 C / -22 F)! We did notice that someone is taking care of them as they have bowls of food about and some cushions here and there – so whomever those angels are, I thank them from the bottom of my heart!

Tomorrow will probably see us getting a few walking tours in :). Tuesday, we do chest x-rays *(compulsory for entering the maternity ward when the time comes – checking for things like TB)*, we have a visit with our surrogate and find out how she and our boys are doing!

More updates soon
Love to you all.
B xxx

Unfortunately, we do have some personal criticisms:

*The housekeeper should have her own room – she sleeps on the sofa bed in the lounge/kitchen. It feels strange as it is having a housekeeper with us all the time, but especially when she doesn't have her own room to go to for privacy (hers and ours). This also means we must vacate the lounge by 10pm and we can't get up in the middle of the night to get something from the kitchen. Although I guess this will be a moot point when the babies are here.

*They don't give us a key for the apartment- this is something that bugged me last time too. So if we want to go out late (obviously before the babies arrive), it means that the housekeeper has to sit up and wait for us. I feel a bit like I'm at my parents' house as a teen.

Here's a summary of the things we learnt about Kyiv today:

*The baby equipment provided in our VIP package should be for twins if the client is having twins. We only have one of everything, so will need to buy additional stuff.

*Wifi signal is pretty crappy.

*Not enough power sockets anywhere around the apartment. This seems to be an Eastern European problem as we encountered this is Czech Republic as well.

Diary Entry 38
One Week Down in Kiev, Ukraine
(about 16 weeks to go)
Published by Bianca on 16 July 2017

Hi Friends!

Thank you to everyone who has been following our surrogacy journey on one of my social media platforms and all those who have sent me personal messages. It's wonderful having you all cheering us on and your excitement for us increases our own excitement! Our little boys are so blessed to already have such amazing people as yourselves in their lives even before they are born! Imagine how loved they will feel when they are old enough to look back and read and understand all your messages and comments. They will never be without love. Thank you all! And so much love back to you!

Well, it's been a week since we arrived in Kiev and what a week it's been! We have had awesome moments mixed with a few not so happy bits but I don't intend to get into that over here. All my gripes and hassles with our clinic are laid out in my surrogacy book, My Ukrainian Surrogacy Journey.

Here's a video link for you with pics highlighting our **Day 2 to 5 in Kiev**
https://youtu.be/O_Xceh7O-5g

The most obvious and the most important part of this week was meeting
our stunning surrogate, getting to know more about our boys through her
and feeling them kick!

She is absolutely divine – gorgeous, glowing with health, the same sense of
humour as Vinny and I (if it wasn't for the difficulty of the language barrier,
I'm sure we would talk every day and become great friends), she has a
happiness & joy that shines from within – such a perfect environment for
our boys to develop in. We could not have chosen anyone better for us. We
are extremely grateful and happy to have her.

We hear from her that our boys love healthy food, especially watermelon.
They are very active and love to box each other (*how typical of Vinny's boys!*)
but they also love dancing (like their mama :)), and when they sleep, they
like to cuddle each other.

She went to start preparations at the maternity hospital this weekend and
we can expect the boys to be born either Monday or Tuesday. Of course,
they could also be stubborn (*their daddy is the most stubborn person I've ever met*)
and decide to keep us waiting for a few weeks still! Either way, the doc said
that they are fully developed and ready to meet us :). Monday is Vinny's
birthday so of course we are hoping for the best birthday present ever! I
have managed to convince the hubster to join me in the delivery room (a
perc of our VIP package with the agency). He's worried about being there,
but I need him to be there for me and stop my own heart from shooting to

the moon with a mix of angst and excitement. I'm in danger of hyperventilating right now just thinking about it!

In other news, we met two lovely couples this week also going through surrogacy in Kiev. One couple (from the UK), we met on Wednesday night for a civilized dinner...well...it was civilized for 3 of us. I won't mention who knocked back a ship load of vodkas. We went to a traditional Ukrainian restaurant where a shot of vodka was less than $1.50 — so how could he resist right?! ha ha! We had a super time with our new friends and look forward to seeing them again.

Friday night we met another couple (from Australia this time) at the Buddha Bar — a popular lounge/nightclub apparently well known for their classy ladies of the night — they were very entertaining. The ladies danced in a harem while an amazing bloke hit his drum non-stop for possibly an hour — he was really good. The sushi was tasty and our Aussie company was awesome. Finally, when the Buddha Bar got too smoky for me to handle (there aren't any no smoking laws in Eastern Europe unfortunately), we moved on to Vinny's favourite playground — a Karaoke Bar — they have hundreds of them in Kiev, at least 5 on every street, all claiming to be 24 hours — Vinny's heaven ha ha! It took a while using Google translate, but he eventually managed to get on the singing list and wasn't too bad — he certainly impressed the ladies (of the night I suspect by the way they jumped all over him with me standing right there! ;). The next day even my eyeballs hurt! We all felt rough, but it was fun!

Despite the way we felt, I still made us get up in the afternoon to make our 90-minute walk into town for food and more baby stuff. We hit a bargain with a changing station, complete with drawers and a bath which can be wheeled around the house for convenience. It was discounted from $350 to under $100. I'm really chuffed with it! It cost about $12 in a taxi to get it home – not bad. The same price as the taxi was at 4am from the Karaoke Bar.

Some other points for the week:

*We are orientating ourselves and getting to know Kiev better each day, doing a lot of walking and discovering new places – especially baby shops, of course! We found another floor of baby and kids shops in a mall called Globus, which is underground of Maiden Square Globus is an upmarket mall with many designer shops.

Excitement is mounting....... the hubby's birthday tomorrow! Could it be Max & Alex's birthdays too?!

Love to you all! xxxx

B & V

Diary Entry 39
Vinny & Bianca's first 10 Days with their newborn sons!
Published by Candice Schwegmann on 05 August 2017

Hello!

My name is Candice Schwegmann. I have recently had the privilege of meeting this phenomenal family and joining them on this journey.

Bianca has allowed me to share on their behalf some highlights of their last few weeks. So, sit, grab some coffee, some tissues and happy reading: –

*Monday 17 July- was Vinny's birthday and they were hoping that the boys would share his birthday. Their surrogate let them know that she was having contractions. After trying to translate her words into something that made sense in English, they concluded that she had Braxton hicks (pre-labour contractions). They tried to do some sightseeing in Kiev but couldn't focus.

*Tuesday 18 July- the parents-to-be tried unsuccessfully to busy themselves while they waited for the news that would change their whole lives. Bianca wishes she could say that they were calm and peaceful, but they couldn't stop themselves from constantly checking if their surrogate was ok and if she needed anything and mostly how long she thought it would be until delivery. She had said all was good and not to worry, that babies would be here that week.

*Wednesday 19 July - more watching and waiting and making sure that they didn't miss THE message. They harassed their surrogate some more to find out how she was and whether they could do anything more to help. At 9.30pm that night they received a long-awaited WhatsApp message from their coordinator to say that their surrogate was in labour and they needed to be on standby. To say they felt a mixture of emotions ranging from excitement to fear and nail-biting nerves, is, to put it mildly. Their clinic coordinator kept vigil with them, ensuring that they did not miss the call from the nurses. However, no call came that night. *Their nerves must have been shattered and even all the way back in sunny South Africa a certain person (me of course!) could have been seen pacing the floors.*

*Thursday 20 July- still no news….at 9am Vinny decided to take a chance and walk to the shop. Of course, shortly afterward they received THE call and Vinny ran at record speed all the way home nearly breaking his ankle! *Murphy's Law…. the poor bloke…* Their driver raced to the hospital. Once there, their translator rushed them around to ensure that they were dressed in the appropriate gear – face masks, overalls and foot covers! They were then whisked into the pre-delivery room where their surrogate was writhing in pain. Bianca felt so sorry for the poor girl – a tiny person carrying these giant boys! Soon some nurses started shouting instructions in Ukrainian that basically related to Bianca, as the intended mother, was the only one allowed in the pre-delivery room and at the birth – Vinny's relief to miss all the gooey stuff of childbirth should be mentioned here! One could just picture this scene – *if it was me, I would have been shouting back in my version of Ukrainian.* Bianca tried to be of some support for their surrogate who "was in definite pain" but she felt so helpless and the language barrier made it even more difficult. She constantly had to use google translate, which by the way was no help at all- so they had to keep phoning the translator.

Bianca said, "It was a strange few hours for all of us but thankfully it was only a few hours before our beautiful boys arrived."

According to Bianca, the birth was an incredible experience. Their surrogate was amazing - no screaming or crying just pushing their boys gently into the world. WOW, what a surreal experience this must have been! Bianca is so happy that she got to be there. *It's something that I am sure she will cherish for her entire life!*

Bianca told me, "Our surrogate was amazing. What an angel! We will always have a special kind of love for her!"

After the birth, they left their boys to get checked out by the doctors and nurses, making sure all the bits and bobs were in place…Vinny had a short glimpse of his little creations, and then they left the hospital in total wonder, disbelief and giddy happiness. Years of disappointments, every failed treatment, every heartache and today they had finally become parents of twin boys! What a moment!

They wanted to go out and celebrate but were just too tired. Instead, they cracked open a bottle of sweet bubbly at home. They are saving a huge bottle of the real thing, a gift from good friends of theirs, for when they are back in Florida celebrating their homecoming. It wasn't long before the exhausted couple fell off into a delightful mix of sleep and a dream…basically a feeling of **"what the eff just happened?"** *I am tempted to tell Bianca and Vinny that they will spend the next couple of years choosing their PJs over going out.*

*Friday 21 July- they found out that the boys had to spend a few days in the hospital. This is apparently a standard procedure for twins in Ukraine even though they were perfectly healthy. Vinny & Bianca set up camp in the hospital on the surrogate wing of the hospital and the nurses brought their boys to them for bonding time.

Bianca said, "The bonding experience was a strange kind of wonderful, frightening and exciting all at once!"

Here's the low down on the new boys:

Maximus Vincent Smith
Born 20 July 2.05pm
Weighing in at 3.430 kg
(7.56 pounds)
Height 54 cm (21 inches)

Alexei Felix Smith
Born 20 July 2.20pm
Weighing in at 3.150 kg (6.94 pounds)
Height 50 cm (19 inches)

The first time they changed a nappy (diaper for the Americans) it took them about 10 minutes- now I am happy to report that according to Bianca they can do it in 10 seconds. That night they both didn': sleep more than an hour- they spent most of their time staring at their boys and making sure that were still breathing!

*Monday afternoon was home day- the boys were discharged, and it was an emotional goodbye with their surrogate. They will see her again in about 6 weeks for parental order paperwork. She was taken home and they were taken to the clinic for DNA tests which is needed for the birth certificates and UK parental order. After all of that, they finally got to their temporary home and set up camp in the lounge/dining room.

They are getting to be a little wiser – a little more experienced – a LOT more tired – and filled with ever-increasing love for their boys.

"It's still difficult not to sob from happiness and gratitude (mixed in with a few tears of exhaustion) when I look at these precious miracles in my arms and our new reality as parents." Bianca says.

They have finally achieved their dream and made a way for their miracle babies and they so look forward to a lifetime of happiness with these two! (*Now I am sobbing…*) I feel really privileged to have been able to share their moments with you and I hope I have relayed their message in the best possible way. Congratulations to this amazing family!!!

All my love
Candice
XO

"That Friday to Monday was a complete haze!!!"

Have a look at the videos that Bianca posted on You Tube shortly after their boys' birth:

Our Twins are 2 hours old

https://youtu.be/ri4UUKt7rvg

Our Twins are 28 hours old

https://youtu.be/7rikcUbHZig

Thanks, from Bianca & Vinny: –

"Thank you so much to every single person who has supported us, stood by us, sent us messages, just been there in some way and helped us to carry on when times were tough and days and nights were too dark to deal with alone. We could not have done it without all of you and you will never know just how grateful we are for having you all in our lives. Thank you from the bottom of my heart and the depths of my soul. And thank you to everyone for sharing in our joy and celebration and for all your happy dances on our behalf. It is so wonderful to have a tribe of amazing people like yourselves in all the really bad times as well as the awesome times – makes everything even more special!! Thank you, thank you, thank you xxxxx
Oceans of love to you!

p.s. Shout out to my hubby, Vinny who has been an absolute model of a perfect dad! I always knew that he would be the best dad, but he has even exceeded my expectations and it makes me beyond happy to see him interact and love our boys the way he does!

 p.p.s. Shout out to all of you who have taken so much of your time to give us tips, suggestions and/or be on the other end of the line when I needed someone to sooth my own tears of helplessness and inexperience.

What they have learned in the 10 first days of being parents

It might not be chocolate balls on the floor – don't pick up it up with bare hands.

Babies love AC/DC (but who doesn't?!).

Little boys pee a lot when the cool air hits their twinkies and you will get hit in the face, mouth, eyeballs, hair and everywhere at least 50 times!

Day/night/mealtimes/showers/brushing teeth/conversations with friends/sleep...all become a big jumbled mess of *not enough*.

Coffee, red bull and chocolate become your best friends every hour of the day.

Another best friend is the baby sounds app…right now the *sssshhhh* sound is doing wonders.

Newborn clothes are made inside out – we thought it was shoddy workmanship at first until we realised that labels and seams can hurt their sensitive skin.

You can never have too many clothes – sometimes they have 3 outfit changes all within one nappy change – little boys!

The best newborn outfits are the ones with the built-in mittens – who would have thought that newborns have such sharp razor blade claws!?! And cutting their miniscule nails is challenging!

They really do grow and change so fast!!!! (Is it crazy that I already feel sad that my little newborns are growing into little infants before my eyes at only 10 days old!?)

Gripe water is another good friend of parents.

What works today to soothe a screaming baby won't necessarily work tomorrow.

You can "watch" a TV program 5 times and still only see 5 seconds of it.

An email can take a week to finish.

Baby poos are exciting – it means that your newborn will be in less pain from gas.

Their personalities are already so distinct from birth!! Our Max has so much character in his eyes and a million different facial expressions. Alex is a little stoner – loves his sleep and is every so chilled!

Life is now divided into nappy (diaper) changes, feeding, soothing, washing clothes, washing and preparing bottles/baby baths and every now and then a stolen few minutes of sleep.

Newborns hiccup and fart a lot ha ha!

Everything one reads in preparation for the arrival of newborns is completely forgotten!

Google is filled with so much contradicting information!! And everyone has a different opinion.

It's insane how many nappies, wet wipes, tissues and formula two babies go through in just a few days!! (our babies strangely only like the pampers wet wipes – all the others make them cry but not pampers – no idea why)

Nappies (at least our brands) have a yellow stripe down the middle that goes blue when wet and need changing. Only found this out recently.

It really was love at first sight and no matter how much they scream and cry for hours, one little look makes your heart melt all over again.

Every day is a baby learning day for babies and parents.

Check out this video of the Twins' first outing in Kiev at 6 days old
https://youtu.be/ho-FLkZOpP8

Diary Entry 40
Our Boys' British Passport Applications are in!
Countdown to leaving Kiev...
Published by Bianca on 05 September 2017

Hi Friends!

Can you believe our twin boys are 7 weeks old already on Thursday?!

We are loving them more than ever! Every day is a new adventure which brings new laughs, smiles and total wonder. It's crazy how much they change and grow daily! They now weigh over four and a half kilos, cry real tears, are trying to play with some of their toys and growing out most of their clothes!

We are still in a state of exhaustion but it's improving now that the boys are on a 4-hour feeding schedule rather than 3 hours.

So yesterday we made application for our boys' British passports. Many of you have been asking whether they will get Ukrainian citizenship as they were born in Ukraine. There aren't that many countries in which people get citizenship simply by virtue of being born in that country – citizenship is usually passed down by the parents and Ukraine is the same. Our boys are British citizens and therefore need to await their British passports before being able to exit Ukraine. Unfortunately for us, this process takes around 10 weeks for a first time British passport and 16 weeks for a first British passport issued to children born via surrogacy. This is a UK (NOT Ukraine) law. After checking the calendar yesterday, I discovered that 16 weeks exactly takes us to Christmas Day!!!

Kiev is already preparing for autumn. Within 2 weeks it has changed from a very hot and sunny 36 degrees C to a grey, misty and somewhat chilly 18 degrees C. The days are getting shorter and the air is getting drier. Soon Florida is going to feel even further away... Please put all those fingers, toes and whiskers together for some speedy passport processing for us – we want the sun and the fresh sea air and to get back to my kitty cats who are missing us so much!

Our Passport experience so far...

*Our babies' Ukrainian birth certificates were issued about 2 weeks after their birth. Our clinic took them for translation and apostille and required final payment before they would release them to us 2 weeks later.

*I emailed the passport application centre with preferred dates and times for our passport application interview (*in our case, this had to be a few weeks later as Vinny was in America*). I received a confirmation email of our date and time the following day.

*We (or rather my husband) spent the next few weeks chasing the clinic for all the required documents. This can get rather time consuming and frustrating, but it won't be done without you constantly on their backs. He put together document files – an originals file and a coloured copies file for each baby, with an index and tabs for ease of reference. I wish he would take this kind of control of every aspect of our lives!! I never realised before that he had the ability to be this organized!!!

*The driver took us (with babies) and our surrogate (with her original identity documents) to our appointment. Our surrogate and I looked after the babies while Vinny went through all the documentation with the official. Total time spent there was around 1.5 hours.

So that's it folks…now we wait and hope that we leave Kiev long before Christmas!

Bye for now!

B xxx

Diary Entry 41
Our Final UK Passport Interview in Kiev is Done
Published by Bianca on 28 October 2017

Hey Friends!

Loads of you have been asking how much longer we will be in Kiev, when we will be home and when they can meet our precious boys! So, here is just a very quick update on how that is going.

We have now been in Kiev for 16 weeks. Our boys are 14 weeks old and Monday will be 8 weeks since our boys' initial passport application. The good news is that Vinny attended our final passport application yesterday and our departure day is very close – finally!

The interview was conducted in a small room with a computer screen and earphones, and Vinny spoke to a lovely lady who sat in a passport office in Sheffield, UK. It was casual and the purpose of the interview was to establish identity and ensure that the boys were really born through legitimate surrogacy and not obtained somehow through the black market. He was asked to confirm random basic facts about himself present and past, including addresses and work, facts about me such as my maiden name and my work, a few facts about the boys and our surrogate. The interview took half an hour and all in all, I understand that it went very well.

The next step is for the interviewer to draw up a report and send it to Belfast where the passports get processed. She could not give Vinny any idea of when we would receive them but did admit that it was a quiet period now, so with luck, things could happen a lot of faster than originally thought – we hope! All fingers and toes crossed for us everyone!

Friends in America, don't get too excited yet though because when we leave Kiev, we still need to travel to the UK to get American visas for the boys which could add on another week or two, but we have a good feeling – just a feeling – that we will be home in Florida before Thanksgiving! The boys' first one.

Lots of love,

B xxx

Oh and HAPPY HALLOWEEN from Maximus & Alexei!

Diary Entry 42
A Kiev Christmas in November – The Twins' Second Photo Shoot
Published by Bianca on 06 November 2017

Hey Friends!

While everyone is waiting for news on our passports and subsequent departure from Kiev, let me tell you about our super fun photo session with our amazing newborn photographer, Vita. We did an Early Christmas shoot and I can't wait to show off the pics!

On Thursday, we went to Goroshynka Photo Studio for a morning of fun for the whole family! Living outside of the city centre, where the roads are virtually impossible to navigate with one baby stroller let alone a double stroller, we are very much confined to our apartment and unless one of the lovely ladies or couples from my Ukraine surrogacy community pop in to visit, we don't get to see any people and are in danger of going completely crazy with cabin fever! It's extremely lonely and boring for all of us, even for the babies! We are on the edge of craziness from people and outing deprivation in our weird little world, shut off from life in general, so any little outing is a great adventure for us!

But, this was not just a little outing. This outing was make-up, dress up and laugh it up with a stunning collection of keepsake photos created by the most talented Vita Sovetova of Sovetoff.photo. Vita is the most beautiful soul – all the babies (and adults) absolutely love her and she is an incredible photographer.

The day started wet, cold, windy – and late! The Über got rather lost on his way to pick us up (*a common occurrence*), so the lovely make-up artist had to work at extra speed to create something decent out of my drowned rat look! Goroshynka studio is one of the largest and impressive in Kiev and it was busy. The boys were so excited to meet new people. They screeched in delight and were full of smiles for everyone. Max enjoyed being the centre of attention as he practiced his tummy time on the studio bed posing like a super star for the camera. Cuteness overload! Both boys did great! They were so good through the costume changes and all the manoeuvring of their little bodies this way and that until they both fell asleep in our arms exhausted!

Speak soon!
B xxx

p.s. keep crossing fingers and toes that we will get our passports any day now!!

Diary Entry 43
Our Surrogate Twin Boys Leave Kiev to Live it up in the UK
Published by Bianca on 19 November 2017

Hi Friends!

Yes, you read the title correctly…the boys finally became British citizens and after 4 months in Kiev, we are finally on our way to pick up our lives again with our new little additions!

First stop – the UK to meet family and friends while we wait for their American visas.

Everything happened quickly!

We received notice that Max & Alex's British passports arrived at the passport centre in Kiev Thursday night. It had been 10 weeks since we made our initial passport application. Friday morning Vinny ran to the centre to get them and what a great feeling to hold those treasured little books in our hands!

We immediately booked our flights to London for Saturday morning and then tackled the huge mountain of packing. It's crazy how much stuff little babies can collect! It was an exhausting task but it was definitely a joyous one! My hubby was amazing. He left me the best job of all - entertaining the cutest babies in the world - while he tried to fit 10 thousand kilos of stuff into two 23 kg bags! Ok, of course it wasn't 10 thousand kilos of stuff. I don't actually know how many kilos it ended up to be, but we had 7 huge bags, each of which was massively overweight, which caused an even bigger confusion for the check-in clerk at the airport, and steam to come out of the ears of the French couple who waited for an hour behind Vinny in the queue while the clerk figured out how to handle this luggage situation!

After a not so VIP experience with our agency in Kiev, we still dared to book the VIP experience at Boryspil airport and I am happy to report that it was indeed a VIP experience I would recommend! For around 200 USD for the family, we had a separate entrance when we arrived at the airport, a personal scanning machine for luggage at both the entrance and before passport control (*we didn't have to take out our laptops, liquids or take off our shoes – what a pleasure!*), an awesome agent that carried all our bags for us from the moment we got there, access to a private family room where we were offered food and drinks as well as a shower in the sparkling bathroom, our own private passport control, a team of lovely, smiling and service-orientated people and a full escort by the agent who carried our hand luggage right up to the doors of the plane – this is extremely helpful when travelling (*especially for the first time*) with twins and no stroller. It was also very helpful when we almost missed the flight due to delays caused by our overstaying in Ukraine. We needed to pay a fine of 850 UAH (32 USD) each for staying for 4 months instead of the permitted 3 months and the processing of this took quite a bit of time, so running to board our plane while each carrying an infant, would have been far more difficult if we didn't have someone carrying our bags! I'm not going to lie, we were shitting ourselves, sweating rivers of anxiety at the thought of delaying our departure any further but the boys were having a fab time looking around, eyes big and alight with curiosity and wonder.

And then we were on the plane, taxing down the runway, and finally in the air with our miracle babies one giant step closer to home! I can't even describe how happy we were! Max sat on Vinny's lap chirping away at the people in their row behind me (*we discovered that for safety reasons, infants from the same family sitting on laps are not permitted to sit next to each other*) and Alex slept all the way on my lap – he didn't even wake up and cry when the pressure bore down on the ears. What little stars we have! We were so proud of them. They were model jet setting babies – which is a good thing, as we have a fair bit of travelling planned over the next year! Thank you to my friends reading this for the baby travel tips :).

I have so much more to tell you about our week, but anyone with twin babies knows that a stolen 10 minutes here and there is all the time us parents have, so long blog posts are going to have to wait until they go to school in a few years. For now, anything outside of twin duty is in bite size chunks, but don't worry, I will fill you in on all our antics as and when I can :).

Right now, we are waiting for their American visas to be processed and issued and then we will be on our way home to Florida. We simply cannot wait!!!!!!

I would love to write more, but this little bit is already taking three days so I will sign off until my next update which will be all about our time in the UK, so watch out for it!

Love to you all from B, Vinny, Alexei & Maximus xxx

Diary Entry 44
Our Twin Boys' First UK Experience
Published by Bianca on 28 November 2017

Hi Friends!

It's been quite a busy time since receiving the boys' passports in Kiev! They have been inundated with new people, sights, sounds, smells, formula, time zones and experiences in the UK and USA. Yes!!! *We are back at home in Florida and feeling AMAZING! The boys have handled everything like the little rock stars they are!*

Here's a summary of our time in the UK:

We arrived on the Saturday morning at Gatwick in London and checked into the airport hotel for the night. While babies hydrated with milk bottles, mama hydrated with a giant G&T & daddy ran around delivering the boys' American visa application to the couriers.

After a hearty English breakfast, we drove 4 hours to Vinny's parents in the north of England. It was the first time that the boys had been in a car seat as Ukraine is not big on health & safety and our agency would not offer us any cars that would fit a car seat. The boys were not fans of the seats and a lot of crying and protesting went on in between feeding and naps.

As soon as we hit Vinny's hometown of Yarm, the craziness began – daily a new group of grandma's friends would stop by to check out the little Vinnies and shower them with a ton of presents and "oohs" and "Aahs". We only just managed to fit in a visit with family and a few of our friends too. The boys were a mix of emotions – excitement and adventure on the one hand and exhaustion and overloading of the brain synapses on the other! They were continuously cuddled, talked to, played with, taken out and introduced to new things (like dogs), which they chose to ignore and the baby bouncer (*the ones that attach to the door frame*) – this was probably the highlight of Max's day!

One of our many highlights, was meeting our friends' girl twins. It was so much fun watching the four them! Alexei was a real lady's man while Max was whiny because he wasn't getting all the attention. Max is an attention hog. Just like my Scruffy Cat, I'm sure he wishes that he was an only child most of the time. But there were times when he and his brother would suddenly notice each other's existence and then the screams of delight and the enormous smiles were to die for! They would look at each other with such amazement and wonder, shutting out the rest of the world. Melts my heart!

I simply loved whizzing around in my iCandy stroller! What a huge difference between the gigantic ship we had in Kiev (*that stroller was seriously longer than a Smart car!*), which I couldn't control at all, to this dainty little iCandy Apple 2 Pear stroller that is brilliant for twins!

At grandma's house, Max discovered his love for a xylophone. We already know that Max loves music (*played loud even*), being sung to by daddy, being danced around by mommy or throwing his hands about to silly nursery rhymes, but his pure joy at seeing and hearing the musical notes of the xylophone put him in a whole different musical category. I'm so excited to see where this will lead.

Also while in the UK, the boys practiced their movements…these would be trying to do some sort of crawling (Alex stretches his arms out like he is swimming and Max lifts his little bottom but doesn't go anywhere yet), sitting up (this is quite funny to see as Max looks like he is doing his daily gym exercises), constant attempts at rolling from back to belly – which eventually paid off for Max as he rolled twice on the last night in the UK – grabbing at toys and the all-important eye-movements…never taking their sights off their bottle of milk!

Other highlights (for dad), was a visit to Saltburn sea. This was not fun for mom as that coast does not have sparkling blue water, sandy beaches or any sort of warm weather. It was brown water, muddy beaches and icy cold winds. Mommy was not impressed. Daddy was proud of his heritage and the boys slept through it all.

The boys also attended their first winter wonderland Christmas display. We were enchanted and overjoyed to finally have kids to take to these Christmassy events (*as everyone who has ever suffered infertility will tell you – Christmas is a hated forced event that is filled with hordes of giggling children and broadly smiling parents that are extra reminders of your failure to produce any of these bubbling beauties*). But this year is different. This year I was the giggling kid bursting with pride as I waltzed around from display to display carrying one of my boys. They seemed mildly interested.

And then 12 days later we were lugging all our oversized bags from the airport hotel to check-in, all the way fending off hordes of fascinated ladies who wanted to look at, touch and find out more about our twins! I felt like I should be doing a singing and dancing show, and well I practically did with my amazing stroller, making this whole business of twinning look easy while dad set about seeing to everything else.

The flight was the emptiest we had been on as everyone else was guzzling down their turkey dinner for Thanksgiving, so with an empty seat between us, no one behind us for the next 15 rows, our babies in bassinets in the bulkhead, we stretched out our legs smugly like we had just won the lottery and dreamed of our homecoming in TAMPA.

Diary Entry 45
Our Kiev-born Twins are finally home in Florida at 4.5 months old
Published by Bianca on 05 December 2017

Hi Friends!

Well, I don't even know where to begin! One minute we were on the plane and the next minute it's 10 days later! It feels amazing to be home! Let me attempt to fill you in on what we have all been up to since our touchdown in Tampa on the night of Thanksgiving 2017.

The boys were as good as gold on the flight and we heard many gasps from passengers as we disembarked. They had no idea there had been 2 babies on board for a 9-hour flight. This got more "*oohs*" and "*aahs*" and "*wow, what good and adorable little babies* ".

They held out through the long march from plane to passport control (we were waved through to the front – one of the many great advantages of having twins :))... they held out during the hour that daddy struggled to gather all 7 huge bags from the luggage belt...they held out while we waited almost another hour for someone to come and help daddy push one of the oversized trolleys while I pushed the stroller… and they held out until daddy left in an Über to collect our car from his office 10 minutes away.

And then it began.…endless screeches and oceans of tears as mommy stood by the pick-up area with all the luggage, rocking Alex in the stroller with one hand and bouncing Max in my free arm while Tampa airport's passengers stared at us wide-eyed – some with sympathy and some with shock. Outwardly I was a proud mama, a picture of calm and control. Inside I felt like an awful mother for running out of formula on the plane – hence why I couldn't feed them then and there. In my defence, this is because we thought that we would be buying on-the-go formula from Boots at Gatwick Airport to take with us, so we didn't bother too much about getting extra beforehand. But they didn't have any formula for us to buy. *What's with you Boots at Gatwick?! This would be where parents travelling with infants would possibly need it the most.*

Finally, daddy arrived with the car and a fresh wave of tears and screams reigned down after being strapped into their new car seats. And these tears and screams lasted 45 minutes from Tampa to St Petersburg where we live. A quick stop at Walmart – daddy tried to soothe cranky, hungry, jet-lagged little munchkins while mommy raced into Walmart dodging the Black Friday queues (*yes, they start already on Thanksgiving night*) in search of formula. I grabbed some ready-to-use off the shelf stuff and hoped for the best (*turned out our boys are not Enfamil fans*). Eventually daddy and mommy were feeding the little ravenous mini Vinnies in the Walmart car park while fending off drunk Thanksgiving well-wishers. Then we were on our way again with only little screams this time.

It felt wonderful to finally walk into our own home, with our own things we are familiar with and love, and specifically my precious little fur babies who ran to me in excitement.

My kitties have been awesome little babysitters! They have been loving the boys, watching over them, coming up to them and kissing their little noses. It's like the kitties have been waiting for these little miracles too! Just perfect! The boys are starting to notice the cats a little here and there and Alex nearly had Scruffy Cat's tail as a teething chew. I'm guessing probably another week or so and they will begin to see the cats as little creatures to interact with.

We dumped all our bags and while daddy made more bottles, mommy introduced Max & Alex to their new Finding Nemo/Lion King room. From the shining eyes and squeals of delight, the room seemed to be a hit. Besides running out of formula, hours of screaming, having no bottle-maker (*we left our Tommee Tippee one in England for return visits*), not having an electric kettle (*it's odd that no one in America seems to have one of these, including us!*), our microwave breaking down within the first 5 minutes of being home (*which meant we were unable to boil water or sterilize bottles*), burning water on the stove top (*yes I know it's unbelievable, but it happened*) and not having space for everything the twins have accumulated over the last 4 months – ***we were overjoyed, ecstatic, blessed and grateful to be back in our home as a family!***

So, what's been happening with the boys since being back?

*They can both *roll continuously* from back to front and front to back again and again.

*They are trying their best to *crawl*.

*Their toys are now much more interesting.

*They are *noticing each other* more.

*They have *attempted food* – green bean puree to be exact. They aren't big fans but will eat it even while pulling funny faces.

Max's musical talent is developing even more as he delights in the drums as well as xylophone.

*They are *sitting up straighter* in the lap and in their new little chair activity centres and intentionally playing with their activity toys.

*They are *trying to sit up all the time* – apparently sitting down is last week's news.

*They are *trying out new sounds* with their tongues, even purposefully imitating the movements of our mouths.

*They are beginning to respond to their own names – although for a moment Alexei thought his name was Monkey Cat Turtle, as that's all we've been calling him for months. He is getting the Alexei idea now ha ha!

*Their *eyes very clearly zone in on their milk bottle* and now the green beans, as well as beer bottles (yes, they are Vinny's boys!).

*Alex has begun *sleeping through the night* – sometimes 6 hours straight – yay more sleep for mommy and daddy!

*They have had a *swim in a real swimming pool* (rather than the bath that they started out swimming in) and they absolutely loved it! They are natural swimmers – a real plus for living in Florida. They have visited the beach and dipped their toes in the Gulf of Mexico – the cold of the water at this time of the year didn't go down too well – their next Gulf swim might have to wait until summer!

*It goes without saying of course that they have been cuddled and played with and wrapped up in attention from everyone they have come across- not just our friends, but strangers have actually stopped their car next to me on our daily walk and jumped out to "ooh" and "aah" over them! I feel like they are celebrities! I'm sure they must feel like they are celebrities too! The bar might be set waaay too high now ha ha!

*We are enjoying daily strolls by the bay and filling up on Florida's (much needed) *vitamin D.*

*They have visited their local paediatrician who confirmed that they are both the picture of health. A BIG picture, weighing in at 16.5 pounds each (around 7.5 kilos), putting them in the 98th percentile for size as well as length!

Right now, we are all just kicking back and enjoying being home as a family in our slice of paradise!

Have a great week everyone!

Speak soon,
B, V, M & A

Diary Entry 46
To the RUDE Stranger who thought it was OK to ask intimate details about my boys' conception…at a Christmas Party!
Published by Bianca on 20 December 2017

Hi Friends!

Before moving on to happier posts, I feel the need to get something off my chest and in doing so provide those who don't know how to handle infertility some ground rules about what is and what is not ok to discuss, ask or refer to with regard to our infertility or children born via IVF / surrogacy.

As we have only been home for less than a month, not many people have seen us and our boys yet, so as you can imagine we have been the talking point of our neighbourhood. Simple walks have turned into photo sessions and a stack of questions from random people, some even stopping their cars to jump out and touch my boys' toes! I now see why I was never awarded any kind of fame, because me and the paparazzi would not have been good mates! While it is very flattering that other people think our babies are as adorable as we think they are, it would be nice for people to enjoy seeing them without interviewing me about every detail of their origin.

Yes, I have always been very open about our infertility experience. Yes, I have shared personal details of our journey to parenthood on a public blog. Yes, I will answer your naturally curious questions (*not a condescending inquest*) about how we finally got our miracle babies if you take me aside and ask whether it is an appropriate moment. However, to meet me at a Christmas party as I arrive into the common area (*especially having never even met before*), to immediately and loudly ask me intimate and probing questions about my fertility, the quality of my eggs, my husband's sperm count, whether we picked up our surrogate from the street and many more questions that totally enraged me at that moment, is more invasive than 4 years of instruments stuck up my hoo ha in front of a room full of doctors. I purposefully tried to deflect the questions, answer vaguely and dismiss the conversation – I was trying to enjoy a Christmas party! But this person ignored my cues and kept pressing and pushing and probing and getting even more personal. *Lady, did you honestly not see the uncomfortable look on my face? Are you not capable of reading body language – mine was trying to block you? Are you generally inconsiderate of other people's privacy and feelings or was it a momentary lapse of politeness, empathy and respect?* And I have some questions for you (lovingly compiled by fellow Fertility Challenged mommies)…

How were your children conceived?
Were you on top or bottom?
Was it a Kama sutra position?
How often do you have sex?
Was it a mistake?

Did the condom break?

Did they cut open your vagina when giving birth?

How is sex now after squeezing out your baby?

How does that feel?! Not very nice when others particularly strangers get into your intimate spaces, is it?

Now, to help you and everyone else who doesn't know how to engage with someone who has fertility challenges or a mother with children after IVF treatments or surrogacy – here are some points to consider:

*There is a *time and place* for these discussions – a party is NOT the time or place.

*Never initiate conversation about how my children were conceived – *I will tell you if I want to*. It is completely up to me to decide whether I would like to speak about personal issues with you or not. Just because I spoke about these things with someone else does not mean I am eager to speak about them to you.

*Always ask me first if I don't mind answering a few personal questions before you take me by surprise.

*This sort of conversation is NOT for a public setting or in front of a group of people unless I'm a guest speaker at a fertility conference!

*At least pretend that you are *interested in getting to know me first* before instantly firing off your questions within seconds of meeting me.

*Never ask how much I paid for our procedures – *accept that it's expensive.*

*Don't ask me if I planned to have twins – *make your own deduction.*

*Don't ask if my children were conceived with my own eggs and my husband's sperm – I cannot even believe people (and by people I mean strangers) have the audacity to ask this question!

*Don't ask me where I "picked up" my surrogate from and if everything about her is healthy or ok – again, how *effing rude*!

*While, I have nothing at all against adoption, surrogacy is not the same thing – so it's best to *get your facts in order* before asking about my "adopted" babies.

*Please do not tell me stories about your aunt's cousin's sister's friend who had fertility issues and then suddenly had a surprise baby – *not relevant to me and I don't care.*

What should you say?
Anything along the lines of…CONGRATULATIONS, WHAT A BLESSING!

Hopefully that will make a good start. I could carry on making a longer list, but I have two gorgeous little boys who need their mommy's attention :). Thank you for listening to me vent! Now that I have emotionally offloaded, hopefully I can move on to simply enjoying being with my beautiful family and celebrate being back home in Tampa with our friends, living and loving this blessed life!
Merry Christmas – Happy Holidays – Blessings for the New Year.

Lots of love,

B (V, A & M)

Diary Entry 47
Our Long Infertility Journey Finally Comes to a Close
Published by Bianca on 20 March 2018

Hi Friends!

Today my boys are 8 months old, which will mark my last blog post on fertility, trying to conceive, IVF and my surrogacy journey. After so many years, it is finally time for me to breathe out all the *trying* and throw myself fully into the *being. Being fully present in the now of motherhood – the place where I have longed to be for over 13 years.*

Thank you so much to every single person who has supported me and my journey, whether it was from day 1 or from yesterday. I appreciate you all and it has only been through this interaction that I was able to keep up my strength and positivity – YOU have gotten me through and there are just not enough words to express how grateful I am to YOU my family, friends, kind strangers and TTC sisters.

Also, thank you to all of you who have supported me in buying either

one or both of my books – I appreciate you too! At the risk of sounding pushy…please leave me a (5 star) review on Amazon. Indie writers like myself rely on as many reviews as we can get for Amazon to spread the word and help us to at least be able to afford a pint of milk with our dry loaf of bread we survive on as writers!

So now that these announcements are done…let me tell you about my AWESOME MARCH!

There were a few not so awesome moments in there – head colds, missing our flight to the UK, exhaustion and dehydration BUT …… **The BEST NEWS, is that WE WERE OFFICIALLY GRANTED A UK PARENTAL ORDER FOR OUR BOYS**….in Vinny's home town (*instead of the usual London High Court*), in one court appearance (*instead of the usual two*) and with no more than an initial Skype consultation with lawyers (*meaning, we saved £20K of the money we would have had to beg someone for*!).

For those not sure what the Parental Order is all about, UK Surrogacy Law declares that the woman who carries and delivers a baby, even when not genetically related to the baby is considered the mother in the eyes of UK law. Once the baby reaches 6 weeks old, procedures can begin for the gestational carrier to relinquish all rights to the baby and for the Intended Parents (us) to be considered the legal parents through many steps and processes, producing detailed statements and evidence in High Court. Even though our boys were born in Ukraine, as we are British, we still need to follow British Law.

Our court appointed case worker scheduled to come and see us on Monday 12th March and our court hearing on **Thursday 15th**. We booked our flights on Virgin Atlantic from Orlando (2 hours away from home) to arrive on Saturday 10th. Our usual flights from Tampa on British Airways were coming in at over $8000 for our dates, so we needed an alternative!

We had it all planned out with a list of things that we would do on schedule and still leave plenty of time to spare for a few relaxing beverages at the airport before boarding our flight. After a whiny night of both boys wrestling imaginary alligators, Alexei woke up the morning of our flight with a very snotty nose – and I do mean the kind of snot that you can make a party load of St Patrick's Day balloons with! Out came the NoseFrida for several sessions with no end to the green slime. We crossed out some not so immediate things on the to-do list in favour of taking the poor boy in to see the doc, wait for test results, wait for meds and then get back to the packing. Incidentally, being a twin mama has severely cut down my personal suitcase to 2 outfits and half the shoes, perfumes and creams I would have taken before the boys arrived, which has kept me coasting at least in the top 5 of the scummy mummy scale! But I digress…

Finally, we were ready to go and only an hour off scheduled time of departure – that would still mean that we would be at the airport 3 hours before our flight and possibly one adult beverage less but still all good.

Ten minutes after leaving home we hit major, almost standstill traffic and this continued for all the 5.5 hours it took us to get to the airport, arriving half hour after our plane had already left! By this time, I had aged 10 years from stress and the boys were hoarse from their screams. It was only toward the end, close to the airport, that we were in a position to stop the car for nappy changes and feeding! It was heart wrenching hearing my babies so distressed and not being able to do anything about it!

In between the howling, I managed a call to Virgin Atlantic's customer service to let them know that we would be missing our flight due to accidents on the highway. With sympathy, the consultant advised that there were only a few seats left for the next day's flight and it would cost around $2100 per adult! We just wanted to cry! As if we hadn't spent enough already! However, the lovely gentleman informed me that there would probably be more passengers missing flights due to the accidents and if that is the case, then we will not be charged the full price of a flight for the next day. I was selfishly crossing things in all sorts of places, that some other poor souls would also miss their flight so that we could be spared spending our boys' non-existent college fund on new flights!

Dehydrated, tired and feeling somewhat defeated by the day, we checked into a tiny room in a Hilton Courtyard in Orlando. The size wouldn't have been too bad if we didn't need to squash two travel cots in between the beds, which the boys absolutely hated. I don't blame them – those things are cold and scratchy and I certainly wouldn't want to sleep in one of those myself! The four of us hardly slept that night. BUT…THE GREAT NEWS was that we were only charged £30 per adult (change fee) for the new flights for the following day!!!!!

Whoop whoop! I wanted to jump through the phone and kiss that Virgin Atlantic consultant and give her my bank card to buy herself something pretty for delivering this super news! Not so super for the people that I hoped would miss their flight too (sorry)…but we needed it! And even better, the flight to London was full so we flew into Manchester which cut our driving travel time by half! Thank you, Universe!

I lay awake waiting for breakfast and despite trying to follow the hubby's footsteps in the Keto diet the previous 2 weeks, I stuffed my face with as many carbs as I could count in 10 minutes! That set me up for NOT digging the eyes out of the security lady made of stone, who didn't stop shouting at Vinny and I to hurry up and get all our stuff through the x-ray machine. She didn't quite grasp that things go a bit slower when you have two infants in arms – Vinny wore Alex and Max was in a little umbrella stroller until that had to be put through the x-ray conveyor machine as well – she shouted this 6 times to me within half a minute. Vinny was ordered to take off his boots which is a challenge while wearing a baby. Stoney b**ch's colleague gave us a look of empathy and words of encouragement before having to take Vinny's shoes off for him!

All this came about shortly after we held up a massive queue of passengers at the Virgin Atlantic check-in because we had forgotten how to collapse our double stroller! All our bags were strewn across all the check-in counters creating a gauntlet for others trying to check-in, Max was doing his best death metal screams, one of the Virgin staff members was trying to fold here and there with Vinny, another was begging us to check how it worked on You Tube and 5 other Virgin Atlantic staff members were playing peekaboo with the boys to calm them down. 6 months ago, I would have begged the floor to open and swallow me to save me from the shame of not having 'it' together. Now with 8-month old twins, having 'it' together means successfully leaving the house with tummies full and nappies changed – or mostly just leaving the house!

The flight was not bad. On the downside, Virgin Atlantic only have the baby bassinets, which my boys have long outgrown, so it wasn't too comfortable for them. British Airways have the bassinets until 6 months old and then they have the car seat style chairs which they fit onto the bassinet tables. On the plus side, we had the full bulkhead row to ourselves, so we could really spread out all our stuff! Also, a huge plus, was the Virgin Atlantic staff. They were superb – genuinely helpful, friendly, really service orientated and they gave the impression that they really did love making us happy – not just doing a job. I cannot thank that aircrew enough for all they did for us, even going as far as offering to carry all our bags to passport control for us. Excellent service all round from them!

We had a wonderful reception of family members come to greet us when we arrived at Vinny's parents' home in Yarm (North East of England). Vinny's mom had put on a huge spread of edible delights and we were spoilt with pressies. It was also Mother's Day in England that day so even though I didn't fully celebrate this first one, it was an added little sweetness for me. The family were so excited to see the boys and the boys were excited to see them – colds and all. Alexei had passed on his snottiness to all 4 of us now with the addition of flaming throats and pounding heads.

Monday, we met with our court appointed case worker and what an angel she is!! Not only is she one of the sweetest people you could ever meet but so kind and considerate and a lady of action. By action I mean that she was fully responsible for arranging our case to be heard in our area instead of London (where it is historically held) and due to her prompt reporting back to the court and boldly requesting the High Court Judge to consider and approve our case all in one sitting due to the logistics of travelling all the way back again, WE WERE AWARDED OUR PARENTAL ORDER ON THURSDAY!!!!!! The Judge (and what a sweetheart he was too!) commended us on our detailed parental order statement to the court, the great organisation of all our documents of evidence and my blog, which he went through before court. It was so good to hear all his fantastic comments and just the best feeling in the world to hear him recording his concluding statement granting us our full legal rights as parents!!! Having never been in a court before, especially in front of a high court judge, this usually outspoken mama lion, became a shy little girl from my nervous energy and could only smile and giggle at the judge stupidly. As soon as he left the room, I burst into happy tears to the amusement of his sweet clerk!

The cherry on the cake, was a stop off at my wonderful friends, Elmarie and Jason. El had helped me to care for the boys in Ukraine for 10 days while Vinny had to fly back to the States for work. They had last seen her when they were 2 months old, but they never forgot. If they had tails, they would have been wagging up a storm from excitement! The reunion melted my heart! They didn't want to leave her. It was the first time that Jason met the boys and they wasted to time in inspecting him eyeball to eyeball and I know J's heart melted too!

All I can say about the 9-hour flight back to Orlando is this – it's going to be a long long long gap before we fly with these two again! Vinny votes age 18 but I'll settle for a few years younger than that. On the other hand, Alexemus (see what I did? He he) made up for their behaviour on the flight by charming absolutely everyone on the way from the plane to our car! These buttery smiles and hypnotic eyes got us directly off the plane, past about 3 hours of waiting in long lines and immediately to the front of passport control!!! That is a total win, especially as we still had a 2-hour drive home. Maybe they just took pity on bedraggled twin parents who had obviously not slept much in months going by their slits for eyes. Whichever it was, it doesn't matter – only that we got ushered to the front in celebrity style. Oh and speaking of celebrities, we even got to the passport counter before Warwick Davis who was on our flight. He looks just the same in person by the way!

All in all – there were so many positives which far outweighed the negatives, so I call that a damn successful trip!

Celebrations this weekend at our place – BBQ, sun, swimming, manatees and dolphins

All is good in our world.

Love B xxx

.

Journey Timeline

Feb 2004 (South Africa):

Stopped taking the contraceptive pill

June 2005:

Various scans and tests by the gynaecologist. Told by gynaecologist and endocrinologist that I needed to be treated for Graves Disease (over-active thyroid) and PCOS.

I was given Clomid (Fertimed in South Africa), Metformin (Glucophage in South Africa) and Carbimazole. (South Africa).

Jan 2006:

Stopped all my meds – personal decision due to the meds making me extremely ill and unable to function from day to day.

Oct 2010 (UK):

Chemical pregnancy – taken to hospital with infection. Various tests and scans.

Confirmed that I did not currently have PCOS.

Jan 2011:

Thyroid tested again and confirmed over-active. Started taking Propylthiouracil (PTU) and monitored every 6 weeks. Was told that fertility treatment could not be started until Thyroid tested normal.

Jan 2012:

Thyroid normal – requested fertility investigations to start.

April 2012:

Day 3 (check ovarian reserve) and Day 21 (progesterone levels to check that ovulation has occurred).

My husband had a semen analysis.

July 2012:

Hysterosalpingogram (HSG) performed to check both tubes – all good.

August 2012:

Referred to a fertility consulting nurse for a 5-minute discussion on what happens next – referred to a fertility specialist.

October 2012:

Repeat of day 3 and day 21 tests.

April 2013:

Repeat of Day 3 test (Serum FSH, Serum LH and Serum TSH).

I was tested for Rubella, HIV, Hepatitis B & C and Chlamydia.

May 2013:

Referred to the fertility specialist at Cotswold Fertility Unit and had to repeat day 3 and day 21 blood tests.

My husband was also tested for HIV and Hepatitis B & C and another semen analysis - ***Normozoospermic (normal).***

June 2013:

Invited to a talk on IVF at Oxford Fertility Clinic.

Haemoglobin test and Serum Ferritin (iron levels).

July 2013:

Met with the fertility planning nurses at Cotswold Fertility Clinic and prepared protocol for first cycle.

Started taking **Buserelin** (Suprecur) down reg sniffing meds (nasal spray every 2 hours) to put my body into forced temporary menopause. Down reg scan to check that ovaries have shut down.

Iron tests showed anaemia – started taking 2 x ferrous sulphate (iron supplements) daily.

August 2013:

Gonal F injections (225ml) to stimulate ovaries to produce as many egg follicles as possible and as large as possible (optimum size between 16 and 21 mm).

Regular scans to check number and size of follicles and decide when they are ready to be harvested.

September 2013:

In danger of over-stimulation (OHSS) so Gonal F reduced to 125ml.

Egg retrieval (9 eggs fertilized).

Cyclogest (progesterone) pessaries – 1x twice a day until pregnancy test.

Day 5 transfer of 2 embryos (1x grade 1 and 1x grade 3) – Lining 8.9mm at time of transfer.

None of good enough quality left over to freeze.

October 2013:

Positive Pregnancy Test.

Early pregnancy scan at 6 weeks and 4 days confirmed one heartbeat.

November 2013:

12-week scan showed that baby's heart had stopped around 8 weeks.

Emergency ERPC (evacuation of retained pregnancy products) performed.

Stopped taking iron tablets.

January 2014:

Follow up with fertility specialist and advised that missed miscarriage was just down to bad luck.

February 2014:

IVF Cycle number 2 begins with **Synarel** down reg sniffing meds (morning and night).

Acupuncture twice a week.

Endo scratch.

March 2014:

Gonal F injections (125ml)

Acupuncture twice a week.

April 2014:

Egg collection (10 eggs fertilized).

Cyclogest (progesterone) pessaries – 1x twice a day until pregnancy test.

Transfer of 2 embryos (2x grade 2) on day 5 of cultivation using Embryo Glue – lining at 10.4mm.

1 embryo to freeze (1x grade 1).

Acupuncture twice a week.

Negative pregnancy test.

May 2014:

Follow up with the fertility specialist – decline in quality of eggs suspected.

June 2014:

IVF Cycle number 3 begins with Synarel

Started taking 1 iron tablet a day.

July 2014:

Gonal F injections (125ml).

August 2014:

Egg collection (5 eggs fertilized).

Cyclogest (progesterone) pessaries – 1x twice a day until pregnancy test.

Transfer of 2 embryos (1x grade 2 and 1x morula) on day 5 – lining at 8.4mm.

None to freeze.

September 2014:

Negative pregnancy test.

October 2014:

Follow up appointment with fertility specialist. She confirmed that egg quality is declining even further. Advised to move on to Egg Donation if our frozen embryo fails to implant.

Second endo scratch.

Started taking one Aspirin (75mg) a day.

November 2014:

Cycle number 4 – natural FET (frozen embryo transfer) using Embryo Glue of our last embryo after natural ovulation confirmed through LH surge home test and scan.

Lining at 7.3mm.

Cyclogest (progesterone) pessaries – 1x twice a day until pregnancy test.

December 2014:

Negative pregnancy test.

Decided to move on to donor eggs in Brno, Czech Republic.

Contacted co-ordinators between us and Reprofit International in Brno. Sent history over and completed all medical and personal forms.

January 2015:

Cycle number 5 begins with Donor Eggs.

Started taking BCP's (birth control pills) to synchronize my cycle with my donor's cycle but had to stop after 5 days as was violently ill – vomiting and migraines – couldn't get out of bed.

Was given Northisterone pills instead of BCP's.

February 2015:
Had down reg injection of **Diphereline** (administered by nurse).

Started **Progynova** estrogen pills.

Scan to check thickness of endometrial lining (6.4mm).

Sperm collection at Reprofit International in Brno, Czech Republic results
as follows:

Volume: 62ml (lowest limits 15ml)
Density: 62 (lowest limits 15)
Motility: 81 (lowest limits 40)
Morphology: 1% (lowest limits 4)
Notes: Teratozoospermia (deformed sperm)

Intralipid infusion.

Started Utrogestan progesterone pessaries on sperm collection day 4x twice a day.

Started taking over-the-counter Vitamin D supplements.

Stopped taking daily Aspirin due to bleeding ulcer.

March 2015:

Lining scan (8.6mm)

Started Utrogestan progesterone pessaries 4x twice a day from sperm collection day.

Transfer of 2 hatching blastocysts on day 5.

Intralipid infusion.

One embryo frozen.

Negative pregnancy test.

Started Progynova oestrogen pills for Cycle number 6 on day 2 of my bleed (which was 5 days after negative test)

April 2015:

Lining scan.

Started taking Prednisone (steroid) pills.

Intralipid infusion 10 days before transfer and on transfer.

Started Utrogestan progesterone pessaries 4x twice a day.

Transfer of our one fully hatched blastocyst which has been frozen.

Steroid injection **Solumedron** administered by nurse after transfer.

Started daily blood thinner injections **Fraxiparine** (Clexane).

Negative pregnancy test.

Started Progynova for Cycle number 7 with PGD CHI Tested Donor Embryo.

May 2015:
Lining scan (6.91mm)

Intralipid infusion 10 days before transfer.

Started Utrogestan progesterone pessaries 4x twice a day.

Transfer of one PGD CHI Tested Donated Embryo. – Lining only 7mm.

NO more intralipids. NO steroid injection. NO more blood thinning injections.

Negative pregnancy test.

June 2015:

Initial consultancy with new clinic called IVI in Barcelona, Spain.

Detailed blood and semen tests done, including various genetic tests.

July 2015:

Results come in for the various tests.

Me: I discover that I have MTHFR homozygous C677T mutation! Treatment for this includes attempts to naturally detox and replace toxic cleaning chemicals and other harmful substances with non-toxic ones. Advised to take Folate (NOT synthetic folic acid) and a complex vitamin B multi-vitamin (NOT pre-natals).

Hubby's Sperm:

Volume: 5 million (lowest limits 1.5million)

Density: 17.05 mill (Lowest limits 15 mill)

Motility: 50 (lowest limits 40)

Morphology: 7% (lowest limits 4)

Notes: Normozoospermia (normal sperm)

FISH genetic test results:

Normal results for the chromosomes analysed (chromosomes 13, 18 and 21).

Started prepping for my ERA test & Hysteroscopy, which included:

2 weeks of birth control – 7 days of cetrotide injections – oestrogen 3 times a day (to thicken the endo lining – progesterone twice a day.

August 2015:

ERA Test & Hysteroscopy (top of uterus concave, which they fixed but that does not affect fertility – everything normal).

September 2015:

ERA results returned – no problems there – my womb is normal and receptive.

Fired IVI Barcelona for lack of professionalism, communication issues, delayed results and repeated mistakes.

Appointed Prague Fertility Centre – perfect egg donor found and genetic testing on her begins to make sure she is not the carrier of the same 5 diseases as Vinny.

October 2015:

Begin birth control pills on day 1 of period to sync my cycle with my donor.

Our donor's genetic testing returned with a positive for carrying one of the same genetic diseases as Vinny – this means that a baby would have 25% chance of being born deaf.

I stop my BCP's and search begins for a new egg donor to retest for the same genetic diseases.

December 2015:

A new donor found, bloods taken and sent to lab for genetic testing.

January 2016:

Begin Northisterone to sync my cycle with donor and be ready for when test results arrive back.

Laparoscopy procedure – **Stage 2 endometriosis** and a small cyst found and removed. We understand that even a small amount of endometriosis can have negative effects on fertility including implantation failure and toxicity to embryos.

Delay in receiving results so I stop Northisterone.

Acupuncture 3 x per week until transfer.

February 2016:

Hubby travels to Prague to give his sperm to freeze. There is a great improvement since his last Sperm Analysis. So, we believe his daily Chinese herbs, pomegranate juice, zinc and copper supplements and very little alcohol has paid off.

Volume: 4 million (lowest limits 1.5million) – this decreases every time but is not essential
Density: 84 mill (Lowest limits 15 mill) – massive improvement
Motility: 69% (lowest limits 40) – great improvement since last SA
Morphology: 5% (lowest limits 4) – this has decreased but still above the line
Notes: Normozoospermia (normal sperm)

Results arrive and whoo hoo – donor is given the all clear!

I start Northisterone 3 times a day to for a week to sync my cycle with donor's.

March 2016

I start Synarel Nasal Spray on CD1 to shut down my ovaries (2 x morn/ 2 x eve for a week then 1 x morn/ 1 x eve for a week)

I also start oestrogen 3 x per day from CD2

CD11: My lining scan shows a great triple layer uterus but only measures 6mm – we need above 7 as a minimum, so my oestrogen has been increased to 5 a day.

Donor's collection was Wed 23 March. She gave 10 eggs, 8 of which fertilised.

I start my progesterone 2 pessaries 3x a day and continue with 5 tabs of oestrogen a day.

Day 5 embryo transfer Mon 28 March – we had 2 embryos left for transfer and 1 to freeze. The embryologist explained that as we were using a young egg donor, there really should have been more healthy embryos by day 5. She said that this indicated a problem with the sperm.

Prescribed Clexane (blood thinner injections) daily.

Test Date: Tuesday 12 April 2016 – NEGATIVE

Exploring Surrogacy

15 October 2016:

First consultation at clinic in Ukraine.

We stayed for a week while Vinny gave 6 samples of sperm to freeze so that we don't have to travel back for egg collection and transfer -only again just before baby's birth.

17 October 2016:

Vinny gave 2 sperm samples and had blood tests taken, we met with our English coordinators, we met with the embryologist, signed the contracts, paid our first instalment and were given access to the database of egg donors (240 ladies!).

19 October 2016:

We made a shortlist of 4 egg donors that we liked and made notes with pros and cons. We then sent this list in the order of our preference to our English-speaking donor/surrogacy coordinator.

2 sperm samples given.

20 October 2016:

We were advised that we had a suitable surrogate and we could either start immediately using our 4th choice in egg donor or wait until our other choices were available. We decided to go with the lady who was immediately available.

2 sperm samples given.

9 November 2016:

Egg donor's retrieval –

9 eggs collected, 8 eggs fertilised, 3 made it to blastocyst – none to freeze

14 November 2016:

3 Grade AA 5-day blastocysts were transferred to our surrogate

28 November 2016:

Surrogate's beta confirmed at 2367!

14 December 2016:

2 strong heartbeats at 6 weeks pregnant! We are expecting twins! Yay!!!!!

31 Jan 2017:

Our twin BOYS are measuring at 13 weeks – due date 7
August 2017!

28 Feb 2017:

Received ultrasound updates on our beautiful boys and they are
doing well. They are measuring between 17 and 18 weeks.

30 March 2017:

Received ultrasound updates on our boys – both looking cuter
and cuter and doing well. They are measuring between 21 and 22
weeks.

28 April 2017:

Our boys are now baking at 26 weeks and getting nice and fat.

31 May 2017:

We met our Surrogate for the first time over skype this morning.
We had a little chat via a translator but both parties were nervous,
and tongue tied. She seemed really sweet, cute and glowing with
health.

Updated scan today, our boys are measuring *30 weeks 2
days* and growing at just over 4 pounds already :)

8 July 2017

We have arrived in Kiev and prepare to welcome our boys, Max & Alex any time soon. Our surrogate is 36 weeks pregnant with them and is getting tired and running out of space. It is estimated on all the IVF due date calculators, that because they are twins, they should arrive around 12 July!!! My hubby guestimates that they will arrive on his own birthday, which is 17 July :). Anything is possible at this stage.

12 July 2017

We had a fantastic visit with our surrogate today. Our boys are fully developed, and our little surrogate's belly is huge. They are ready to make an appearance any day now.

18 July 2017

Our surrogate starts contractions.

20 July 2017

Our sons, Maximus Vincent Smith and Alexei Felix Smith were born!!!

24 July 2017

The boys get discharged from the hospital with complete health!

4 September 2017

Applied for the boys' British passports after 9 weeks in Kiev.
Could be here anything from another 6 to 16 weeks! 16 weeks
takes us to exactly Christmas Day!

27 October 2017
Final British passport interview. Now we wait for the passports to
be printed and sent to us!

6 November 2017
Passport office in Belfast confirmed that our passports have been
printed and that we would receive them in 7 to 10 working days.

09 November 2017
We received word that our passports are ready for collection.

10 November 2017
We collected our passports from the local passport centre

11 November 2017
We finally left Kiev and flew to the UK to apply for our boys'
American visas

23 November 2017
We arrived back home in Tampa!

15 March 2018

Awarded official UK Parental Order, our long fertility journey ends and our family adventures continue.

ABOUT THE AUTHOR

At the time of writing, Bianca Smith is a 44-year-old, South African-born IVF veteran, having done 8 IVF transfers between 2013 and 2016. She currently lives in Tampa, Florida where she is loving life with her British-born husband, Vinny, two cats, Fatty & Scruffy and twin boys, Maximus Vincent Smith & Alexei Felix Smith, born 20 July 2017, through the blessing of surrogacy in Ukraine.

She has two previous fertility books available on Amazon:

IVF A Detailed Guide and My Ukrainian Surrogacy Journey

HAVE YOU ENJOYED THIS BOOK?

If you have enjoyed this book, I would be very grateful if you would post a short and positive review on Amazon. Your support really does make a difference to me!